CONTENTS

ECG/EKG Interpretation

Complete Handbook for 12-Lead ECG Interpretation and the Diagnosis and Management of Arrhythmias

DR. AALIYAH RAMDEEN

TEKHEALTH
TECHNOLOGY IS YOUR HEALTH

Dr. Aaliyah Ramdeen

Complete Handbook for 12-Lead ECG Interpretation and the Diagnosis and Management of Arrhythmias

Editors

Dr. Marcus B. Antoine

Dr. Nia Baptiste

ISBN: 978-5-4241-6028-8

Tek Health

Printed in the United States of America

INTRODUCTION

Electrocardiogram (ECG/EKG) interpretation is an essential skill in the field of cardiology, playing a crucial role in diagnosing and managing heart conditions. This comprehensive guide aims to equip healthcare professionals with a thorough understanding of 12-lead ECG/EKG analysis and the methods for diagnosing and treating arrhythmias.

An ECG/EKG records the electrical activity of the heart, providing valuable insights into its function and rhythm. By interpreting these recordings, healthcare providers can identify abnormalities such as arrhythmias, myocardial infarctions, and other cardiac disorders. Mastery of ECG/EKG interpretation involves recognizing normal patterns, as well as deviations that indicate pathology.

The 12-lead ECG/EKG is a standard tool in clinical practice, offering a detailed view of the heart's electrical activity from multiple angles. Each lead captures information from different parts of the heart, enabling a comprehensive assessment. Understanding the significance of each lead, the placement of electrodes, and the typical waveforms is fundamental to accurate interpretation.

Arrhythmias, or irregular heartbeats, can range from benign to life-threatening. This guide covers the various types of arrhythmias, their characteristics on an ECG/EKG, and the underlying mechanisms. Effective diagnosis is crucial for determining the appropriate treatment, which may include medications, lifestyle changes, or medical procedures such as ablation or the implantation of a pacemaker.

Additionally, this guide delves into advanced topics such as interpreting ECG/EKG changes in different clinical scenarios, including electrolyte imbalances, ischemia, and hypertrophy. It also addresses common pitfalls and challenges in ECG/EKG interpretation, providing strategies to overcome them.

By the end of this guide, readers will have a solid foundation in 12-lead ECG/EKG analysis and arrhythmia diagnosis, empowering them to make informed clinical decisions and improve patient outcomes. Whether you are a seasoned practitioner looking to refresh your knowledge or a student beginning your journey in cardiology, this comprehensive guide serves as an invaluable resource for mastering ECG/EKG interpretation.

PURPOSE OF ECG/EKG

The purpose of an ECG/EKG is multifaceted, encompassing various aspects of heart health management. Primarily, it is used to diagnose heart conditions by detecting and evaluating irregularities in the heart's electrical activity, which can indicate issues such as arrhythmias, heart attacks, and other cardiac disorders. It is a crucial tool for monitoring heart health, allowing healthcare professionals to track the progression of heart conditions and assess the effectiveness of treatments.

Additionally, an ECG/EKG is essential for evaluating symptoms that may be related to heart problems, such as chest pain, palpitations, dizziness, and shortness of breath. This helps in determining whether these symptoms are due to cardiac issues. It is also a standard procedure in preoperative assessments, ensuring that a patient's heart health is stable enough for surgery and identifying any potential risks that could arise during the procedure.

Routine checkups often include ECG/EKGs, especially for individuals with a history of heart disease or those at risk of developing cardiac conditions. This regular monitoring helps in the early detection and management of heart problems, contributing to overall cardiovascular health. In summary, an ECG/EKG is a vital diagnostic and monitoring tool in the field of cardiology, aiding in the assessment, diagnosis, and management of heart-related conditions.

IMPORTANCE IN CLINICAL PRACTICE

In clinical practice, the ECG/EKG plays a pivotal role as a diagnostic tool for assessing cardiac health. It provides critical information about the heart's electrical activity, aiding in the detection and characterization of various heart conditions. By interpreting ECG/EKG results, healthcare providers can diagnose arrhythmias, ischemic heart disease, myocardial infarction, and other cardiac abnormalities promptly and accurately. This diagnostic capability allows for timely interventions and personalized treatment plans, improving patient outcomes and reducing the risk of complications. Moreover, ECG/EKG monitoring is essential for assessing the effectiveness of cardiac medications, guiding therapeutic decisions, and monitoring patients during critical care settings. Its widespread use underscores its indispensable role in modern cardiology and clinical care.

BASIC PRINCIPLES OF ECG/EKG

The ECG (electrocardiogram), also known as EKG (electrocardiography), is a cornerstone of cardiovascular diagnostics in clinical practice. It functions by detecting and recording the electrical impulses generated by the heart during each heartbeat cycle. These impulses are crucial as they initiate and coordinate the heart's muscle contractions, ensuring effective pumping of blood throughout the body.

In practical terms, the ECG/EKG involves placing electrodes on specific points of the body's surface, typically on the chest, arms, and legs. These electrodes detect the small electrical changes on the skin caused by the heart's electrical activity. The recorded signals are then amplified and displayed as a series of waveforms on graph paper or a digital screen.

Each wave on the ECG/EKG tracing represents a different electrical event in the heart's cycle:

- P wave: Represents atrial depolarization, which precedes atrial contraction.
- QRS complex: Indicates ventricular depolarization, leading to ventricular contraction.
- T wave: Marks ventricular repolarization, where the heart muscle prepares for the next contraction.

The intervals and segments between these waves provide insights into the heart's rhythm, rate, and the conduction pathway of the electrical impulses. Abnormalities in these patterns can indicate various cardiac conditions, such as arrhythmias, myocardial ischemia, electrolyte imbalances, and structural heart diseases.

In clinical practice, the ECG/EKG serves several critical purposes:

1. Diagnosis: It aids in diagnosing a wide range of cardiac disorders by identifying abnormal electrical patterns or changes indicative of specific conditions.

2. Monitoring: Continuous or intermittent ECG/EKG monitoring helps track the progression of heart conditions, assess treatment effectiveness, and detect new abnormalities.

3. Screening: Routine ECG/EKG screenings are valuable for identifying asymptomatic heart conditions or risk factors, facilitating early intervention and prevention.

4. Prognosis: ECG/EKG findings contribute to assessing the severity and prognosis of cardiac conditions, guiding appropriate management strategies.

5. Research: ECG/EKG data are essential in clinical research, providing insights into cardiac physiology, disease mechanisms, and treatment outcomes.

Overall, the ECG/EKG's fundamental principles of detecting and interpreting cardiac electrical activity play a pivotal role in cardiovascular medicine, offering valuable diagnostic, prognostic, and therapeutic insights that inform patient care and management strategies.

UNDERSTANDING THE 12-LEAD ECG/EKG

Understanding the 12-Lead ECG/EKG involves interpreting the heart's electrical activity through a detailed analysis of twelve different perspectives. This diagnostic tool helps healthcare professionals identify abnormalities in the heart's rhythm, detect heart attacks, and monitor overall cardiac health. It's crucial for diagnosing and managing various cardiovascular conditions, providing valuable insights into the heart's functioning and guiding appropriate treatment decisions.

OVERVIEW OF THE 12-LEADS

The 12-lead ECG/EKG is a crucial diagnostic tool in cardiology that offers a detailed assessment of the heart's electrical activity. Unlike a single-lead ECG, which provides a limited view, the 12-lead ECG records electrical signals from twelve different perspectives or "leads" across the chest and limbs. Each lead measures the electrical impulses traveling through the heart from a specific angle, allowing healthcare providers to evaluate the heart's performance comprehensively.

This multi-lead approach enables the identification of various cardiac conditions by analyzing the timing and pattern of electrical signals. For instance, it can reveal abnormalities such as arrhythmias (irregular heartbeats), myocardial infarctions (heart attacks), conduction disorders, and hypertrophy (enlargement) of the heart muscle.

Healthcare providers use the 12-lead ECG/EKG in several clinical settings:

- Diagnostic Tool: It helps diagnose acute and chronic cardiac conditions by detecting abnormalities in the heart's electrical system.
- Monitoring: Continuous monitoring with 12-lead ECG assists in tracking changes in cardiac function over time, especially in critical care settings or during procedures.
- Treatment Guidance: It guides treatment decisions by providing insights into the effectiveness of medications, pacemakers, or other interventions.
- Risk Assessment: By assessing electrical patterns, healthcare providers can evaluate the risk of future cardiac events and make informed decisions about patient management.

Overall, the 12-lead ECG/EKG is indispensable for cardiologists, emergency physicians, and other healthcare professionals involved in cardiac care. Its ability to provide a comprehensive overview of heart function significantly contributes to accurate diagnosis, timely intervention, and improved patient outcomes.

LEAD PLACEMENT AND CONFIGURATION

Lead Placement and Configuration in ECG/EKG is crucial for accurately capturing and interpreting the heart's electrical activity. The placement of electrodes, or leads, follows a standardized protocol to ensure consistent and reliable readings across different patients and healthcare settings.

Limb Leads

Limb leads are named I, II, III, aVR, aVL, and aVF. These leads are placed on the arms and legs:

- Lead I: Positioned between the right arm (RA) and left arm (LA).
- Lead II: Positioned between the right arm (RA) and left leg (LL).
- Lead III: Positioned between the left arm (LA) and left leg (LL).
- aVR: Placed on the right arm (RA).
- aVL: Placed on the left arm (LA).
- aVF: Placed on the left leg (LL).

These limb leads provide a view of the heart's electrical activity in different frontal plane axes, allowing for the assessment of electrical vectors moving towards or away from each lead.

Chest Leads

Chest leads, also known as precordial leads, include V1 to V6. These leads are placed on specific locations across the chest wall:

- V1: Positioned at the 4th intercostal space just right of the sternum.
- V2: Positioned at the 4th intercostal space just left of the sternum.
- V3: Placed between V2 and V4.
- V4: Positioned at the 5th intercostal space mid-clavicular line.
- V5: Placed horizontally at the same level as V4 in the anterior axillary line.
- V6: Positioned horizontally at the same level as V4 and V5 in the mid-axillary line.

These chest leads provide a view of the heart's electrical activity in the horizontal plane, allowing for the assessment of electrical vectors moving anteriorly and posteriorly across the chest.

By strategically placing these electrodes according to standardized anatomical landmarks, healthcare providers can obtain a comprehensive view of the heart's electrical activity from different perspectives. This approach facilitates accurate diagnosis and monitoring of various cardiac conditions, including arrhythmias, myocardial infarction (heart attack), and other abnormalities in cardiac rhythm and conduction.

CHAPTER 1

BASICS OF ECG/EKG

An ECG (electrocardiogram) or EKG is a test that records the electrical activity of the heart over a period of time using electrodes placed on the skin. This test is essential for diagnosing and monitoring heart conditions.

The heart's electrical system controls the heartbeat by generating and conducting electrical signals. These signals cause the heart muscles to contract and pump blood. The main components of this system are the sinoatrial (SA) node, atrioventricular (AV) node, bundle of His, right and left bundle branches, and Purkinje fibers.

An ECG/EKG waveform consists of several key parts:

a. P Wave: Represents atrial depolarization, which initiates the contraction of the atria.
b. QRS Complex: Indicates ventricular depolarization, leading to the contraction of the ventricles. It includes the Q wave (initial negative deflection), R wave (first positive deflection), and S wave (subsequent negative deflection).
c. T Wave: Represents ventricular repolarization, the recovery phase after ventricular contraction.
d. U Wave: Occasionally seen following the T wave, its origin is less well understood but may be related to repolarization of the Purkinje fibers or interventricular septum.

Other important intervals and segments include the PR interval, which measures the time for the electrical impulse to travel from the SA node to the ventricles, and the ST segment, representing the period when the ventricles are depolarized.

Understanding these basic components helps in identifying normal versus abnormal heart rhythms and detecting various cardiac conditions such as arrhythmias, conduction abnormalities, and myocardial infarction.

CARDIAC ELECTROPHYSIOLOGY

Cardiac electrophysiology is the study of the electrical properties and activities of the heart. Understanding these principles is fundamental to interpreting ECG/EKG tracings accurately. The heart's ability to generate and propagate electrical impulses is what ultimately results in its rhythmic contractions, pumping blood throughout the body. Here, we will delve into the key aspects of cardiac electrophysiology, including the structure of the heart's conduction system, the generation of electrical impulses, and how these impulses are represented on an ECG/EKG.

ELECTRICAL CONDUCTION SYSTEM OF THE HEART

The heart's ability to function effectively as a pump depends on its electrical conduction system. This system generates and transmits electrical impulses that coordinate the contraction of the heart muscle, ensuring efficient blood flow. Understanding the electrical conduction system is crucial for interpreting ECG/EKG tracings and diagnosing various cardiac conditions.

Components of the Conduction System

1. Sinoatrial (SA) Node

- Location: The SA node is located in the right atrium near the opening of the superior vena cava.
- Function: Known as the heart's natural pacemaker, it generates electrical impulses at a rate of 60-100 beats per minute (bpm) under normal conditions. These impulses initiate each heartbeat.

- Role in ECG/EKG: The electrical activity originating from the SA node causes the P wave on the ECG/EKG, representing atrial depolarization.

2. Atrioventricular (AV) Node

- Location: The AV node is situated in the interatrial septum, near the tricuspid valve.
- Function: The AV node acts as a gatekeeper, slowing down the electrical impulse before it passes to the ventricles. This delay ensures that the atria have enough time to contract and empty their blood into the ventricles before ventricular contraction begins.
- Role in ECG/EKG: The delay in the AV node is reflected in the PR interval on the ECG/EKG, which represents the time taken for the impulse to travel from the atria to the ventricles.

3. Bundle of His (AV Bundle)

- Location: The Bundle of His extends from the AV node into the interventricular septum.
- Function: It conducts the electrical impulses from the AV node to the right and left bundle branches.
- Role in ECG/EKG: The Bundle of His is not directly visible on the ECG/EKG, but its function is crucial for the timing and propagation of the QRS complex.

4. Right and Left Bundle Branches

- Location: These branches run along the interventricular septum.

- Function: They carry the electrical impulse to the right and left ventricles, respectively.
- Role in ECG/EKG: The activity of the bundle branches contributes to the formation of the QRS complex, which represents ventricular depolarization.

5. Purkinje Fibers

- Location: These fibers form a network spread throughout the ventricles.
- Function: Purkinje fibers distribute the electrical impulse throughout the ventricles, ensuring coordinated and rapid contraction.
- Role in ECG/EKG: Their activity is integral to the QRS complex, ensuring that ventricular depolarization occurs efficiently.

Phases of the Cardiac Cycle in Relation to ECG/EKG

1. Atrial Depolarization (P Wave)

- Initiation: The SA node generates an impulse.
- Propagation: The impulse spreads through the atria, causing atrial contraction and pushing blood into the ventricles.
- Representation on ECG/EKG: The P wave indicates atrial depolarization.

2. Atrioventricular Delay (PR Interval)

- Conduction: The impulse travels from the atria to the AV node, where it is delayed. This delay allows for complete ventricular filling.

- Representation on ECG/EKG: The PR interval, measured from the onset of the P wave to the start of the QRS complex, indicates the time the impulse takes to travel through the atria, AV node, and the initial part of the ventricular conduction system.

3. Ventricular Depolarization (QRS Complex)

- Initiation: The impulse travels through the Bundle of His, bundle branches, and Purkinje fibers.
- Propagation: The impulse spreads rapidly through the ventricles, causing them to contract and pump blood to the lungs and the rest of the body.
- Representation on ECG/EKG: The QRS complex represents ventricular depolarization. It is a sharp, tall wave due to the rapid and synchronized electrical activity in the ventricles.

4. Ventricular Repolarization (T Wave)

- Recovery: The ventricles recover from depolarization, preparing for the next cycle.
- Representation on ECG/EKG: The T wave represents ventricular repolarization, where the ventricles reset electrically and get ready for the next contraction.

Clinical Significance

Understanding the electrical conduction system of the heart is essential for diagnosing and managing various cardiac conditions. Abnormalities in this system can lead to arrhythmias, which are deviations from the normal heart rhythm. Here are some common examples:

1) Sinus Bradycardia: A slower-than-normal heart rate due to reduced activity of the SA node.
2) Atrioventricular Block: A delay or blockage of electrical impulses as they travel from the atria to the ventricles.
   - First-Degree AV Block: Characterized by a prolonged PR interval, indicating a delay in conduction through the AV node.
   - Second-Degree AV Block (Type I and II): Intermittent failure of some impulses to be conducted through the AV node. Type I is characterized by progressively lengthening PR intervals until a beat is dropped, while Type II involves sudden dropped beats without a change in the preceding PR intervals.
   - Third-Degree AV Block: Complete failure of impulses to be conducted from the atria to the ventricles, leading to a complete dissociation between atrial and ventricular activity.
   - Bundle Branch Block: A delay or blockage of electrical impulses in the right or left bundle branches, resulting in a widened QRS complex and altered ventricular contraction.

Practical Application in ECG/EKG Interpretation

When interpreting an ECG/EKG, a systematic approach is essential. This involves assessing the following:

1. Heart Rate: Calculated by measuring the intervals between R waves.

2. Heart Rhythm: Determined by evaluating the consistency of P waves and their relationship to QRS complexes.

3. Axis Deviation: Assessed by looking at the overall direction of the electrical activity in the heart.

4. P Wave Morphology: Examined for signs of atrial enlargement or other abnormalities.

5. QRS Complex Morphology: Analyzed for signs of ventricular hypertrophy, bundle branch blocks, or other conduction abnormalities.

6. ST Segment and T Wave Morphology: Checked for signs of ischemia, infarction, or electrolyte imbalances.

The electrical conduction system of the heart is a sophisticated and essential network that ensures the timely and coordinated contraction of the heart muscle. By understanding its components and their functions, healthcare professionals can interpret ECG/EKG tracings accurately. This knowledge allows for the diagnosis and treatment of various cardiac conditions, ensuring effective clinical practice and improved patient outcomes.

GENERATION OF THE ECG/EKG SIGNAL

The heart's electrical activity originates in the sinoatrial (SA) node, located in the right atrium. This node is often referred to as the heart's natural pacemaker because it generates electrical impulses that initiate each heartbeat. The conduction pathway includes the following key structures:

1. Sinoatrial (SA) Node:

- Located in the right atrium near the opening of the superior vena cava.
- Generates electrical impulses at a regular rate, typically 60-100 beats per minute in a healthy adult.
- These impulses cause atrial contraction, which pushes blood into the ventricles.

2. Atrioventricular (AV) Node:

- Located at the junction of the atria and ventricles.
- Acts as a gatekeeper, delaying the impulse slightly before passing it to the ventricles. This delay allows the ventricles to fill with blood from the atria.

3. Bundle of His:

- A collection of heart muscle cells specialized for electrical conduction.
- Transmits the impulses from the AV node to the ventricles.

4. Right and Left Bundle Branches:

- Divisions of the Bundle of His that run along the interventricular septum.

- Conduct impulses to the right and left ventricles, respectively.

5. Purkinje Fibers:

- Network of fibers that spread throughout the ventricles.
- Conduct the impulse rapidly to ensure coordinated contraction of the ventricles, allowing efficient ejection of blood.

Generation of the ECG/EKG Signal

The ECG signal is generated by the flow of ionic currents across the myocardial cell membranes during the different phases of the cardiac cycle. This activity is recorded by electrodes placed on the skin surface.

Ionic Currents and Action Potentials

Cardiac muscle cells, or myocytes, generate action potentials due to the movement of ions across their cell membranes. The primary ions involved are sodium (Na+), potassium (K+), and calcium (Ca2+). The action potential of a cardiac cell consists of several phases:

1. Phase 0 (Depolarization):

- Rapid influx of Na+ ions through fast sodium channels.
- Causes the cell membrane potential to rise sharply, initiating the contraction.

2. Phase 1 (Initial Repolarization):

- Na+ channels close.
- Brief outflow of K+ ions.

3. Phase 2 (Plateau Phase):

- Ca2+ channels open, allowing calcium ions to enter the cell.
- Balances the outflow of K+, leading to a plateau in the action potential.

4. Phase 3 (Repolarization):

- Ca2+ channels close.
- Continued outflow of K+ returns the cell to its resting membrane potential.

5. Phase 4 (Resting Phase):

- The cell is at its resting membrane potential, maintained by the Na+/K+ pump.
- The cell is ready to be depolarized again by the next electrical impulse.

The ECG Waveform

The electrical activity of the heart is captured as a series of waves and intervals on the ECG. These components reflect the depolarization and repolarization of different parts of the heart:

1. P Wave:

- Represents atrial depolarization.
- Occurs when the SA node triggers an electrical impulse, causing the atria to contract.

2. QRS Complex:

a. Represents ventricular depolarization.
b. Consists of three distinct waves:

- Q Wave: The initial negative deflection.
- R Wave: The first positive deflection.
- S Wave: The negative deflection following the R wave.
- Ventricular contraction follows the QRS complex.

3. T Wave:

- Represents ventricular repolarization.
- Occurs as the ventricles prepare to return to their resting state.

4. U Wave (if present):

- Represents the repolarization of the Purkinje fibers or papillary muscles.
- Not always visible and its significance is often debated.

Intervals and Segments

Intervals and segments on the ECG provide additional information about the timing and duration of cardiac events:

1. PR Interval:

- Measured from the beginning of the P wave to the beginning of the QRS complex.
- Reflects the time taken for the electrical impulse to travel from the SA node through the AV node and into the ventricles.

2. QRS Duration:

- The time taken for ventricular depolarization.
- Measured from the beginning of the Q wave to the end of the S wave.

3. QT Interval:

- Measured from the beginning of the QRS complex to the end of the T wave.
- Represents the total time for ventricular depolarization and repolarization.

4. ST Segment:

- Measured from the end of the S wave to the beginning of the T wave.
- Represents the period between ventricular depolarization and repolarization.

The generation of the ECG signal is a complex process involving the orchestrated activity of the heart's electrical conduction system and the ionic movements across cardiac cell membranes. By interpreting the ECG waveform, healthcare providers can assess the electrical and mechanical functions of the heart, diagnose arrhythmias, and identify other cardiac abnormalities. Understanding the fundamentals of ECG signal generation is crucial for accurate interpretation and effective clinical decision-making.

COMPONENTS OF THE ECG/EKG WAVEFORM

The components of the ECG/EKG waveform are fundamental elements that healthcare professionals analyze to assess cardiac health and diagnose various conditions.

P WAVE

The P wave in an electrocardiogram (ECG/EKG) represents the depolarization of the atria. It is the first positive deflection seen on the ECG tracing and signifies the electrical activity that stimulates atrial contraction. Here's a comprehensive explanation of the P wave:

The P wave is a small, typically rounded waveform that precedes the QRS complex on the ECG.

Its characteristics include:

a) Shape and Duration: Normally, the P wave is smooth and upright, lasting approximately 0.06 to 0.11 seconds (60 to 110 milliseconds) in duration.
b) Origin: The P wave originates from the depolarization of the atria, specifically from the sinoatrial (SA) node, the natural pacemaker of the heart. This depolarization spreads through the right and left atria, causing them to contract and pump blood into the ventricles.
c) Interpretation: Clinically, the P wave provides essential information about the atrial depolarization and the conduction pathway through the atria. Changes in the P

wave morphology can indicate abnormalities such as atrial enlargement, atrial hypertrophy, or conduction delays within the atria.

d) Measurement: Important measurements related to the P wave include its amplitude (height) and duration. Changes in these measurements can provide insights into the health of the atria and the conduction system.
e) Clinical Correlations: Abnormalities in the P wave can indicate conditions such as atrial fibrillation (absence of a distinct P wave), atrial flutter (sawtooth appearance of P waves), or atrioventricular (AV) block affecting the conduction from the atria to the ventricles.

Understanding the P wave is crucial in interpreting the overall rhythm of the heart and diagnosing various cardiac arrhythmias. It serves as a fundamental component in assessing the electrical activity of the atria and its contribution to overall cardiac function.

QRS COMPLEX

The QRS complex in an electrocardiogram (ECG/EKG) represents the depolarization of the ventricles of the heart. It is a crucial component of the ECG waveform and provides essential diagnostic information about the heart's electrical activity.

Anatomy of the QRS Complex

The QRS complex consists of three distinct waves:

a) Q Wave: This is the initial downward deflection from the baseline. It represents depolarization of the interventricular septum.

b) R Wave: The R wave is a positive deflection following the Q wave. It signifies depolarization of the main mass of the ventricles.
c) S Wave: The S wave is a negative deflection following the R wave. It indicates the completion of ventricular depolarization or depolarization of the septum opposite to where the Q wave appears.

Characteristics and Interpretation

a) Duration: The duration of the QRS complex is normally between 0.06 to 0.10 seconds (60 to 100 milliseconds). Prolongation may indicate conduction delays or blockages within the ventricles.
b) Amplitude: The amplitude of the QRS complex reflects the amount of electrical activity generated during ventricular depolarization. Abnormalities in amplitude can indicate hypertrophy (enlargement) or infarction (damage) of the heart muscle.

Clinical Significance:

a) Normal QRS Complex: In a healthy heart, the QRS complex is typically uniform in shape and duration.
b) Abnormalities: Various conditions can alter the appearance of the QRS complex, including bundle branch blocks (delayed conduction in one of the main branches of the heart's electrical system), electrolyte imbalances (such as hyperkalemia or hypokalemia), and myocardial infarction (heart attack).

Diagnostic Use

a) Localization of Damage: Specific changes in the QRS complex, such as ST segment elevation or pathological Q waves, can help localize areas of myocardial damage in conditions like myocardial infarction.
b) Arrhythmias: Analysis of the QRS complex helps diagnose and classify different types of arrhythmias, such as ventricular tachycardia and bundle branch blocks.

The QRS complex is a fundamental part of ECG interpretation, providing insights into the electrical activity of the ventricles. Understanding its characteristics and variations is essential for diagnosing cardiac conditions and guiding clinical management.

T WAVE

The T wave is a crucial component of the electrocardiogram (ECG/EKG) waveform, representing the ventricular repolarization phase of the cardiac cycle. It follows the QRS complex, which signifies ventricular depolarization.

The T wave on an ECG/EKG graphically represents the electrical activity associated with the recovery, or repolarization, of the ventricles. This phase begins as the ventricles start to relax and prepare for the next contraction.

Key points about the T wave include:

- Timing and Duration: The T wave typically follows the QRS complex, appearing as a smooth, rounded wave that returns the ventricles to their resting state electrically. Its duration is normally less than 0.2 seconds.

- Shape and Morphology: A normal T wave is usually upright in leads where the QRS complex is upright (like leads I, II, V3-V6) and inverted where the QRS complex is inverted (such as aVR and aVL). The shape and amplitude can vary based on factors such as heart rate, electrolyte balance, and medications.

- Interpretation: Clinicians interpret the T wave to assess for abnormalities that may indicate conditions such as myocardial ischemia, electrolyte disturbances (e.g., hyperkalemia or hypokalemia), myocardial infarction, or drug effects (e.g., digitalis toxicity). Abnormalities include flattening, inversion, or tall, peaked T waves.

- Clinical Relevance: In clinical practice, evaluating the T wave is crucial for diagnosing and monitoring various cardiac conditions. Changes in T wave morphology or presence of abnormal T waves can provide valuable diagnostic clues and guide treatment decisions.

Understanding the T wave in the context of the entire ECG/EKG allows healthcare providers to assess cardiac health, detect abnormalities early, and formulate appropriate management strategies to optimize patient care.

U WAVE (IF PRESENT)

The U wave is a small, typically positive deflection that may appear after the T wave in some electrocardiograms (ECGs/EKGs). It is not always present and is most commonly seen in leads V2 and V3, though it can appear in other leads as well. The U wave is usually subtle, following the T wave closely, and often merges with it, making it challenging to distinguish at times.

The exact physiological origin of the U wave is not fully understood, but several theories exist:

- Repolarization Phase: It is believed to represent the late repolarization phase of the Purkinje fibers or papillary muscles.

- Electrolyte Imbalances: Changes in electrolyte concentrations, particularly hypokalemia (low potassium levels), can accentuate the U wave.

- Drugs and Medications: Certain medications, such as digoxin, antiarrhythmics (e.g., Class IA and III), and electrolyte-altering drugs, may cause or exaggerate the U wave.

The clinical significance of the U wave is not as well-established as other ECG waves. In some cases, a prominent U wave can be associated with hypokalemia or other electrolyte disturbances. However, its presence alone does not necessarily indicate pathology. Clinicians typically interpret the U wave in context with the entire ECG and the patient's clinical history.

In essence, while the U wave is a recognized component of the ECG/EKG waveform, its interpretation requires careful consideration of other ECG features, clinical context, and potential influencing factors such as electrolyte levels and medications.

INTERVALS AND SEGMENTS

In ECG/EKG interpretation, understanding intervals and segments is crucial for assessing cardiac function and identifying abnormalities. These components provide valuable insights into the timing and coordination of electrical events within the heart.

PR INTERVAL

The PR interval on an ECG/EKG represents the time it takes for the electrical impulse to travel from the atria (specifically, the sinus node) to the ventricles. It is measured from the beginning of the P wave to the beginning of the QRS complex. This interval includes the time it takes for the impulse to travel through the atria, the AV node, the bundle of His, and the bundle branches before spreading to the ventricular myocardium.

The normal duration of the PR interval typically ranges from 0.12 to 0.20 seconds (3 to 5 small squares on standard ECG paper, each representing 0.04 seconds). This interval is crucial as it reflects the time necessary for the atria to depolarize and for the impulse to be transmitted through the AV node and the His-Purkinje system to initiate ventricular contraction.

An abnormally prolonged PR interval (greater than 0.20 seconds) can indicate various conditions, such as first-degree heart block, where the impulse conduction through the AV node is delayed but every impulse is still conducted to the ventricles. Conversely, a shortened PR interval (less than 0.12 seconds) may suggest pre-excitation syndromes like Wolff-

Parkinson-White (WPW) syndrome, where there is an abnormal accessory pathway allowing early ventricular depolarization.

Understanding the PR interval is essential in diagnosing and evaluating different cardiac conditions, providing insights into the conduction system's functionality and potential abnormalities affecting cardiac rhythm and efficiency.

QRS DURATION

In ECG/EKG interpretation, the QRS duration refers to the time it takes for the electrical impulse to travel through the ventricles of the heart. It is measured from the beginning of the Q wave to the end of the S wave in the QRS complex. This duration is clinically significant as it provides insights into various cardiac conditions.

A normal QRS duration typically ranges from 0.06 to 0.10 seconds (60 to 100 milliseconds) in adults. This duration can vary based on age, sex, and individual differences, but deviations outside this range may indicate underlying cardiac abnormalities.

Clinical Significance

- Normal QRS Duration: A normal QRS duration indicates that the electrical impulse is conducting normally through the ventricles. This suggests that the depolarization process within the ventricles is proceeding as expected.

- Prolonged QRS Duration (QRS Widening): This may be indicative of conduction delays within the ventricles, often associated with conditions such as bundle branch blocks (e.g., Right Bundle Branch Block (RBBB), Left Bundle Branch Block (LBBB)) or ventricular conduction delays. It can also occur in conditions like myocardial infarction, electrolyte imbalances, or certain medications affecting conduction.

- Shortened QRS Duration: A shortened QRS duration is less common but may occur in conditions such as Wolff-Parkinson-White (WPW) syndrome or ventricular tachycardia, where there is rapid conduction through an abnormal pathway.

Interpretation

Interpreting QRS duration involves comparing the measured duration with normal values and considering the clinical context. It is crucial in diagnosing and managing various cardiac arrhythmias and conduction abnormalities. In clinical practice, QRS duration is assessed alongside other ECG parameters to understand the overall electrical activity of the heart and guide treatment decisions.

QT INTERVAL

The QT interval on an ECG/EKG represents the duration of ventricular depolarization and repolarization. It starts at the beginning of the QRS complex and ends at the end of the T wave. This interval is crucial as it reflects the time taken for the ventricles to contract and then reset electrically for the next contraction.

Key Points about the QT Interval:

- Measurement: The QT interval is measured from the beginning of the QRS complex to the end of the T wave. It is typically corrected for heart rate (QTc) using formulas like Bazett's formula ($QTc = QT / \sqrt{RR \text{ interval}}$).

- Normal Duration: In adults, a normal QT interval is generally considered to be less than 0.44 seconds (440 milliseconds), though this can vary slightly depending on age, gender, and heart rate.

- Clinical Significance: Prolongation of the QT interval can predispose individuals to a type of arrhythmia called Torsades de Pointes, which can degenerate into ventricular fibrillation and sudden cardiac death. Causes of QT prolongation include medications (e.g., antiarrhythmics, certain antibiotics), electrolyte imbalances (e.g., hypokalemia, hypocalcemia), and congenital syndromes (e.g., Long QT syndrome).

- Shortened QT Interval: A shortened QT interval is less common but can occur in conditions such as hypercalcemia or as a result of certain medications.

- Assessment: When interpreting an ECG/EKG, it's important to assess the QT interval in relation to the patient's overall clinical context and any concurrent medications or electrolyte abnormalities. This evaluation helps determine whether further investigation or intervention is necessary to mitigate the risk of dangerous arrhythmias.

Understanding the QT interval and its variations is critical for healthcare professionals in diagnosing and managing patients with cardiac conditions or those at risk of arrhythmias.

ST SEGMENT

The ST segment is a crucial part of the electrocardiogram (ECG/EKG) waveform that represents the period between ventricular depolarization (completion of the QRS complex) and the beginning of ventricular repolarization (onset of the T wave).

It is a flat, isoelectric line on the ECG tracing that occurs immediately after the QRS complex and before the T wave.

Key Characteristics of the ST Segment:

- Duration and Timing: Typically, the ST segment should be flat and should not deviate from the baseline (isoelectric line). It usually lasts from the end of the S wave to the beginning of the T wave.

- Measurement: Clinicians measure the ST segment at the J point, which is the junction between the QRS complex and the ST segment. Any deviation from the baseline at this point can indicate myocardial injury or ischemia.

- Elevation: ST segment elevation refers to a rise above the baseline level of the ECG tracing. This elevation can be significant if it is greater than 1 mm (0.1 mV) in two or more contiguous leads. ST segment elevation is typically associated with acute myocardial infarction (heart attack) or pericarditis.

- Depression: ST segment depression refers to a downward deflection from the baseline level of the ECG tracing. It is significant if it is greater than 0.5 mm (0.05 mV) in two or more contiguous leads. ST segment depression can indicate myocardial ischemia, especially when it occurs during exercise or stress testing.

Clinical Significance

- Myocardial Ischemia: ST segment changes (elevation or depression) are crucial indicators of myocardial ischemia. Ischemia causes an imbalance between myocardial oxygen supply and demand, leading to changes in the ST segment.

- Myocardial Infarction: Persistent ST segment elevation (greater than 1 mm in contiguous leads) is a hallmark of acute myocardial infarction (AMI). It indicates ongoing damage to the myocardium due to coronary artery occlusion.

- Other Conditions: Aside from ischemia and infarction, ST segment changes can also occur in conditions such as pericarditis (where there is diffuse ST segment elevation) and myocarditis.

Interpretation

Interpreting ST segment changes requires a systematic approach, considering the patient's clinical context, symptoms, and other ECG findings. It's important to correlate these changes with the patient's history and other diagnostic tests (such as cardiac enzymes and imaging studies) to determine the underlying cause accurately.

In summary, the ST segment on an ECG/EKG provides critical information about myocardial electrical activity and is a key indicator of myocardial ischemia or injury. Understanding its normal appearance and recognizing deviations from the baseline are essential skills in clinical practice for diagnosing and managing cardiac conditions.

CHAPTER 2

INTERPRETING THE 12-LEAD ECG/EKG

Interpreting the 12-Lead ECG/EKG is a fundamental skill in clinical practice, crucial for assessing cardiac health and diagnosing various heart conditions. A 12-lead ECG/EKG provides a snapshot of the heart's electrical activity from multiple angles, using electrodes placed on specific locations on the body.

Each lead in the 12-lead ECG/EKG represents a different perspective of the heart's electrical activity. By comparing the electrical signals recorded from these leads, healthcare providers can evaluate the rhythm, rate, and morphology of the cardiac cycle.

1. Key Aspects of Interpreting a 12-Lead ECG/EKG

- Lead Placement and Configuration: Understanding where each lead is placed on the body and how they relate to the heart's position is crucial. Leads are classified into limb leads (I, II, III, aVL, aVR, aVF) and precordial leads (V1-V6), each capturing electrical signals from specific areas of the heart.

a) Waveform Analysis

The ECG/EKG waveform consists of several components:

- P Wave: Represents atrial depolarization.
- QRS Complex: Indicates ventricular depolarization.

- T Wave: Shows ventricular repolarization.
- ST Segment and QT Interval: Evaluated for abnormalities that may suggest ischemia, injury, or electrolyte imbalances.

b) Rate and Rhythm: Determining the heart rate (beats per minute) and assessing the regularity of the heart rhythm (sinus rhythm, atrial fibrillation, etc.) are critical initial steps in interpretation.

c) Axis Determination: Calculating the electrical axis of the heart helps identify deviations that could indicate chamber enlargement or conduction abnormalities.

d) Morphological Analysis: Analyzing the shape, duration, and amplitude of waves and complexes across different leads provides insights into specific cardiac conditions such as hypertrophy, ischemia, or infarction.

e) Clinical Correlation: Integrating ECG/EKG findings with patient history, symptoms, and other diagnostic tests enhances accuracy in diagnosis and management decisions.

2. Challenges in Interpretation

- Artifact Recognition: Differentiating between true cardiac signals and artifacts caused by patient movement or improper electrode placement.
- Variant Presentations: Recognizing normal variants in ECG/EKG patterns across demographics, as well as pathological conditions that alter typical waveforms.

- Dynamic Changes: Understanding how ECG/EKG findings can change over time, particularly in response to interventions or evolving clinical conditions.

3. Clinical Utility

- Diagnostic Tool: Primary for diagnosing arrhythmias, ischemia, myocardial infarction, and electrolyte imbalances.
- Monitoring Tool: Continuously assessing cardiac function during procedures, anesthesia, and critical care settings.
- Screening: Identifying risk factors and early signs of cardiac abnormalities, even in asymptomatic individuals.

Interpreting the 12-lead ECG/EKG requires proficiency in waveform recognition, systematic analysis, and clinical correlation to provide accurate assessments and guide effective patient care.

SYSTEMATIC APPROACH TO ECG/EKG INTERPRETATION

The systematic approach to ECG/EKG interpretation is crucial for healthcare providers to accurately assess cardiac rhythm and identify potential abnormalities.

This methodical analysis involves several key steps that ensure a comprehensive evaluation of the electrocardiogram (ECG/EKG):

1. Rate and Rhythm Assessment

a) Heart Rate: Begin by calculating the heart rate, which is essential for understanding cardiac function. Count the number of QRS complexes in a 6-second strip and multiply by 10 to determine beats per minute (bpm). Normal adult heart rate ranges from 60 to 100 bpm.

b) Rhythm: Determine if the rhythm is regular or irregular. Regular rhythms have consistent intervals between QRS complexes, whereas irregular rhythms exhibit variation in QRS intervals. Irregular rhythms may indicate atrial fibrillation, atrial flutter, or other arrhythmias.

2. P Wave Analysis

Examine the P waves in each lead. Normal P waves are smooth, upright, and typically precede every QRS complex. Abnormalities in P wave morphology, such as absence or variation in shape, can indicate atrial enlargement, conduction abnormalities (like atrioventricular block), or ectopic atrial rhythms.

3. PR Interval Measurement

Measure the PR interval, which extends from the beginning of the P wave to the beginning of the QRS complex. Normal PR interval duration ranges from 0.12 to 0.20 seconds (3-5 small squares on ECG paper). A prolonged PR interval (>0.20 seconds) suggests first-degree atrioventricular block or other conduction delays, while a shortened PR interval (<0.12 seconds) may indicate pre-excitation syndromes (e.g., Wolff-Parkinson-White syndrome).

4. QRS Complex Evaluation

Assess the QRS complex for duration and morphology. Normal QRS complex duration is typically less than 0.12 seconds (3 small squares). Wide QRS complexes (>0.12 seconds) can indicate bundle branch blocks (left or right) or ventricular conduction delays. The morphology of the QRS complex should be evaluated for abnormalities such as tall or broad complexes, which may suggest ventricular hypertrophy or conduction abnormalities.

5. ST Segment Analysis

Examine the ST segment, which follows the QRS complex and precedes the T wave. Normally, the ST segment is isoelectric (flat) and located at the baseline. Elevations or depressions of the ST segment may indicate myocardial ischemia, injury (such as acute myocardial infarction), or pericarditis. The ST segment should be measured at the J point, the junction between the QRS complex and the ST segment.

6. T Wave Assessment

Evaluate the T waves for morphology and symmetry. Normal T waves are usually upright and rounded in most leads. Inverted, peaked, or flattened T waves can indicate myocardial ischemia, electrolyte disturbances (such as hyperkalemia), or other cardiac conditions.

7. Axis Determination

Determine the electrical axis of the heart, which reflects the overall direction of ventricular depolarization. Axis deviation may indicate chamber enlargement (left or right) or conduction abnormalities. Axis deviation can be assessed by examining the QRS complexes in leads I and aVF.

8. Clinical Correlation and Further Assessment

Consider the patient's clinical history, symptoms, and additional diagnostic tests (such as echocardiography or stress testing) to corroborate ECG/EKG findings. Integrated assessment helps differentiate between benign variants and clinically significant abnormalities, guiding appropriate management and treatment decisions.

By employing a systematic approach to ECG/EKG interpretation, healthcare providers can effectively diagnose arrhythmias, ischemic heart disease, conduction abnormalities, and other cardiac conditions. This structured method ensures thorough evaluation and enhances patient care by facilitating timely interventions and management strategies based on accurate diagnostic information.

RATE

In electrocardiography (ECG or EKG), the rate refers to the number of heartbeats per minute (bpm) as measured from the ECG tracing. It is a fundamental aspect of ECG interpretation and provides crucial information about cardiac rhythm and function.

Understanding Rate in ECG/EKG

The rate can be determined by several methods:

- Counting Method: In a paper ECG, the rate can be calculated by counting the number of QRS complexes (or R waves) in a standard time interval (usually 6 seconds) and multiplying by 10 to get beats per minute.

- Measuring R-R Interval: For irregular rhythms, measuring the time between successive R waves (R-R interval) and calculating the rate based on the average interval.

- Automated Measurement: Modern ECG machines often provide automated calculations of heart rate, which are based on the duration between successive R waves.

Clinical Significance of Rate

- Normal Heart Rate: In adults, a normal resting heart rate ranges typically from 60 to 100 bpm. Rates below or above this range may indicate bradycardia (slow heart rate) or tachycardia (fast heart rate), respectively.

- Rate Variability: Rate variability can provide insights into autonomic nervous system function and overall cardiovascular health. It can be influenced by factors such as age, fitness level, medications, and stress.

Interpretation Considerations

- Determining Regularity: The regularity of heart rate (whether it is regular or irregular) is crucial in diagnosing arrhythmias. Regular rhythms have consistent intervals between QRS complexes, while irregular rhythms vary in interval duration.

- Clinical Context: Interpreting heart rate in the context of symptoms and clinical history is essential. For instance, a patient presenting with palpitations may have a tachyarrhythmia, whereas a patient with dizziness and fatigue may have bradyarrhythmia.

Practical Application

- Assessment of Treatment Response: Monitoring heart rate changes during treatment (e.g., with antiarrhythmic medications) helps assess the effectiveness of therapy.

- Monitoring During Procedures: Continuous ECG monitoring during procedures and surgeries helps detect immediate changes in heart rate, guiding clinical decision-making.

In summary, heart rate interpretation in ECG/EKG provides critical information about cardiac rhythm, helping clinicians diagnose and manage various cardiovascular conditions. Understanding the methods of rate calculation, its clinical significance, and interpretation considerations are essential for accurate ECG/EKG analysis and patient care.

RHYTHM

In ECG/EKG interpretation, "rhythm" refers to the pattern and regularity of the heart's electrical activity as recorded on the tracing. It is determined by the sequence of cardiac depolarization and repolarization events, which control the contraction and relaxation of the heart muscles.

Key aspects of rhythm analysis include:

- Regularity: Evaluating whether the intervals between consecutive heartbeats (R-R intervals) are consistent.
- Rate: Calculating the heart rate, typically by counting the number of QRS complexes in a given time frame.
- P Wave Consistency: Checking if each QRS complex is preceded by a P wave, indicating that the heartbeat is initiated by the sinoatrial (SA) node.
- PR Interval: Measuring the time between the onset of the P wave and the start of the QRS complex to assess atrioventricular (AV) conduction.
- QRS Duration: Ensuring the duration of the QRS complex is within the normal range, indicating proper ventricular depolarization.

AXIS

In ECG/EKG interpretation, the axis refers to the overall direction of the electrical activity of the heart as it propagates through the ventricles. This is typically assessed using the frontal plane leads (leads I, II, III, aVL, aVR, and aVF) to determine the heart's mean electrical vector during ventricular depolarization, primarily observed in the QRS complex.

Normal Axis

1. A normal QRS axis falls between -30° and +90°.
2. The electrical vector points downward and to the left, reflecting the typical pathway of ventricular depolarization.

Left Axis Deviation (LAD)

1. An axis between -30° and -90°.
2. This can be due to conditions like left ventricular hypertrophy, left bundle branch block, or inferior myocardial infarction.

Right Axis Deviation (RAD)

1. An axis between +90° and +180°.
2. Often associated with right ventricular hypertrophy, right bundle branch block, or pulmonary conditions like chronic obstructive pulmonary disease (COPD).

Extreme Axis Deviation (No Man's Land)

1. An axis between -90° and ±180°.
2. Rare and often indicates severe conduction abnormalities or ventricular rhythms.

Determining the Axis

Lead I and Lead aVF Method:

1. Look at the QRS complexes in leads I and aVF.
2. If both are positive, the axis is normal.
3. If Lead I is positive and aVF is negative, check Lead II; if Lead II is positive, it's a normal axis; if negative, it indicates LAD.
4. If Lead I is negative and aVF is positive, it's RAD.

5. If both Lead I and aVF are negative, it's extreme axis deviation.

Understanding the axis is essential in diagnosing and identifying underlying cardiac or systemic conditions that may alter the heart's electrical activity.

P WAVE MORPHOLOGY

The P wave on an ECG/EKG represents the electrical depolarization of the atria, which precedes the contraction of the atria. Analyzing the morphology (shape, size, and appearance) of the P wave is essential for diagnosing various cardiac conditions, particularly those related to atrial activity.

Normal P Wave Characteristics

- Shape: The P wave should be smooth and rounded.

- Duration: The normal duration is less than 0.12 seconds (less than three small squares on the standard ECG grid).

- Amplitude: The height of the P wave should be less than 2.5 mm in the limb leads (such as leads I, II, and III) and less than 1.5 mm in the precordial leads (such as V1 and V2).

- Direction: The P wave is usually positive (upward) in leads I, II, aVF, and V2 to V6, and it is typically biphasic (having both a positive and negative component) in lead V1.

Abnormal P Wave Morphology

- P Mitrale: This is characterized by a P wave with a notched or "m-shaped" appearance, often seen in lead II. It indicates left atrial enlargement, typically due to conditions like mitral valve disease.

- P Pulmonale: This refers to a tall, peaked P wave, often greater than 2.5 mm in height in lead II, indicative of right atrial enlargement, commonly associated with pulmonary hypertension or chronic lung disease.

- Inverted P Waves: Inverted P waves in leads where they are normally upright (such as leads II, III, and aVF) suggest an ectopic atrial rhythm, where the atrial impulse originates outside the SA node, or a retrograde conduction from the AV junction.

- P Waves in Atrial Fibrillation: In atrial fibrillation, distinct P waves are absent. Instead, there are irregular, fibrillatory waves due to chaotic atrial activity.

- P Waves in Atrial Flutter: Atrial flutter produces a "sawtooth" pattern of flutter waves, particularly visible in the inferior leads (II, III, aVF), with a regular atrial rate usually around 250-350 beats per minute.

Clinical Significance

- Atrial Enlargement: Abnormal P wave morphology can indicate atrial enlargement or hypertrophy. For instance, a P mitrale suggests left atrial enlargement, while a P pulmonale suggests right atrial enlargement.

- Atrial Ectopic Activity: Inverted or abnormal P waves can indicate atrial ectopic rhythms, where the electrical impulses originate outside the SA node.

- Conduction Abnormalities: Variations in P wave morphology can provide clues about atrial conduction pathways and the presence of conduction blocks.

Understanding the P wave morphology is fundamental in diagnosing and managing various cardiac conditions, as it provides insight into atrial function and potential underlying pathologies.

QRS COMPLEX MORPHOLOGY

The QRS complex represents ventricular depolarization, which is the process by which the ventricles of the heart are electrically activated to contract and pump blood. Analyzing the morphology of the QRS complex is essential in understanding the electrical activity of the heart, diagnosing various cardiac conditions, and assessing the overall function of the ventricles.

Components of the QRS Complex

- Q Wave: The initial negative deflection before the R wave. It represents depolarization of the interventricular septum. A normal Q wave is typically small and narrow. Pathological Q waves, which are wider and deeper, may indicate a previous myocardial infarction.

- R Wave: The first positive deflection after the Q wave. It reflects the main mass of the ventricles being depolarized. The R wave amplitude varies depending on the lead and the individual's heart anatomy.

- S Wave: The first negative deflection after the R wave. It represents the final depolarization of the ventricles, particularly the base of the heart.

Normal QRS Complex Characteristics

- Duration: A normal QRS complex duration is less than 0.12 seconds (120 milliseconds). A duration longer than this may indicate a conduction delay or block.

- Amplitude: The amplitude of the QRS complex varies across different leads but generally should not exceed 2.5 to 3.0 millivolts in the limb leads. Tall R waves may suggest left ventricular hypertrophy, while low voltage QRS complexes can be seen in conditions like pericardial effusion or obesity.

- Axis: The QRS axis, which represents the overall direction of the heart's electrical activity during ventricular depolarization, typically ranges from -30° to +90° in a normal heart. Deviations in the axis can indicate conditions such as left or right ventricular hypertrophy or conduction abnormalities.

Abnormal QRS Complex Morphologies

1. Bundle Branch Blocks (BBB):

- Right Bundle Branch Block (RBBB): Characterized by a QRS duration > 0.12 seconds and a pattern of RSR' (a second R wave) in the right precordial leads (V1 and V2). This indicates delayed activation of the right ventricle.

- Left Bundle Branch Block (LBBB): Also has a QRS duration > 0.12 seconds with broad, notched R waves in the left precordial leads (V5 and V6) and deep S waves in the right precordial leads (V1 and V2). This indicates delayed activation of the left ventricle.

2. Ventricular Hypertrophy:

- Left Ventricular Hypertrophy (LVH): Often presents with increased QRS amplitude in the left-sided leads (e.g., V5, V6) and deep S waves in the right-sided leads (e.g., V1, V2). The Sokolow-Lyon criteria (S wave in V1 + R wave in V5 or V6 > 35 mm) is commonly used to diagnose LVH.

- Right Ventricular Hypertrophy (RVH): May show tall R waves in the right precordial leads (V1, V2) and deep S waves in the left precordial leads (V5, V6).

3. Myocardial Infarction (MI):

- Pathological Q waves and changes in the R wave progression across the precordial leads can indicate an old or evolving MI. ST segment changes often accompany acute MI, but persistent Q waves may be a marker of an old infarction.

4. Pre-excitation Syndromes:

- Conditions like Wolff-Parkinson-White (WPW) syndrome feature a short PR interval and a delta wave (a slurred upstroke of the QRS complex), indicating an accessory pathway.

5. Additional Considerations

- Fragmented QRS Complexes: Fragmented QRS complexes (presence of additional R waves or notching of the R or S waves) can indicate areas of myocardial scar or fibrosis, often seen in ischemic heart disease.

- Poor R Wave Progression: Normally, the R wave amplitude should increase from V1 to V6. Poor R wave progression, where this increase is not observed, can be a sign of anterior myocardial infarction or other anterior wall abnormalities.

Understanding the QRS complex morphology provides crucial insights into the electrical activity and structural condition of the heart, aiding in the diagnosis and management of a wide range of cardiac disorders.

ST SEGMENT AND T WAVE MORPHOLOGY

The ST segment in an ECG/EKG represents the period between ventricular depolarization and repolarization. It starts at the end of the QRS complex (the J point) and ends at the beginning of the T wave.

Normal ST Segment:

In a healthy heart, the ST segment is usually isoelectric, meaning it lies flat along the baseline of the ECG. However, slight deviations can occur and may still be considered normal. It's important to evaluate the ST segment in the context of the overall clinical picture and ECG findings.

ST Segment Elevation:

Elevation of the ST segment can be a sign of acute myocardial infarction (heart attack). When significant (typically more than 1-2 mm in contiguous leads), it suggests injury to the heart muscle. This elevation is often associated with a convex or upward shape but can also present as concave or saddle-shaped, depending on the underlying cause.

Other causes of ST segment elevation include:

- Pericarditis: Typically presents with diffuse ST elevation across multiple leads and is often concave.
- Early repolarization: A benign condition seen mostly in young, healthy individuals.
- Left ventricular hypertrophy or bundle branch block: Secondary to these conditions rather than primary myocardial injury.

ST Segment Depression:

ST segment depression is usually a sign of ischemia, indicating that part of the heart muscle is not getting enough blood flow. This can occur in conditions such as:

- Stable angina or non-ST elevation myocardial infarction (NSTEMI)
- Digitalis effect: A down-sloping ST depression known as the "scooped" ST segment.
- Reciprocal changes in the setting of ST elevation myocardial infarction.

T Wave Morphology

The T wave represents ventricular repolarization, the process by which the heart's ventricles return to their resting state. T wave morphology can provide important clues about the heart's electrical activity and overall health.

Normal T Wave:

In most leads, the T wave is upright. It is usually smooth and asymmetrical, with a slower upstroke and a faster downstroke. In lead V1, the T wave can be variable, and in some healthy individuals, it may be inverted.

T Wave Inversion:

Inverted T waves can indicate several pathological conditions, including:

- Myocardial ischemia: Often seen in leads corresponding to the affected area.
- Previous myocardial infarction: Indicative of past damage, especially if accompanied by pathological Q waves.
- Ventricular hypertrophy: Due to increased myocardial mass.
- Bundle branch blocks: Often associated with changes in T wave morphology.
- CNS events (e.g., stroke or intracranial hemorrhage): Can cause diffuse T wave inversions.

Peaked T Waves:

Tall, peaked T waves are often a sign of hyperkalemia (high potassium levels). They can be a critical finding requiring urgent treatment to prevent life-threatening arrhythmias. Peaked T waves can also be seen in the early stages of myocardial infarction.

Flattened T Waves:

Flattened T waves can suggest hypokalemia (low potassium levels) or other electrolyte disturbances. They may also occur in conditions of increased vagal tone.

Biphasic T Waves:

T waves that go in one direction and then change direction are known as biphasic T waves. This can be seen in:

- Myocardial ischemia: Biphasic T waves, particularly in the precordial leads, can indicate a high risk of significant coronary artery disease.
- Hypokalemia: Can also produce biphasic T waves.

Clinical Importance

Accurate interpretation of the ST segment and T wave morphology is crucial in diagnosing and managing various cardiac conditions. Changes in these components can provide early warning signs of myocardial infarction, ischemia, and other critical conditions. However, it's important to consider the clinical context, patient history, and other ECG findings when interpreting these changes.

DETERMINING HEART RATE

Determining the heart rate from an ECG/EKG is a fundamental skill in cardiology and is crucial for assessing cardiac function. The heart rate indicates how many times the heart beats per minute (bpm). There are several methods to calculate the heart rate from an ECG/EKG, each with its own advantages. Here are the most common methods:

The 300 Method

The 300 method is a quick and straightforward way to estimate the heart rate. This method is useful when the rhythm is regular.

1. Identify an R Wave on a Bold Line: Locate an R wave that falls on a bold line (large box).

2. Count the Large Boxes Between Two R Waves: Count the number of large boxes between this R wave and the next R wave.

3. Calculate the Rate: Divide 300 by the number of large boxes. The formula is:

$$\text{Heart Rate (bpm)} = \frac{300}{Number\ of\ Large\ Boxes\ Between\ R\ Waves}$$

For example, if there are 4 large boxes between R waves, the heart rate is:

$$\frac{300}{4} = 75\ bpm$$

The 1500 Method

The 1500 method is more precise and is also used for regular rhythms.

1. Count the Small Boxes: Count the number of small boxes between two consecutive R waves.

2. Calculate the Rate: Divide 1500 by the number of small boxes. The formula is:

$$\text{Heart Rate (bpm)} = \frac{1500}{Number\ of\ Large\ Boxes\ Between\ R\ Waves}$$

For instance, if there are 20 small boxes between R waves, the heart rate is:

$$\frac{1500}{20} = 75\ bpm$$

The 6-Second Method

The 6-second method is commonly used for irregular rhythms, but it can be used for regular rhythms as well.

1. Mark a 6-Second Interval: On the ECG/EKG strip, identify a 6-second interval. This is typically marked by 30 large boxes (each large box is 0.2 seconds, so 30 large boxes equal 6 seconds).

2. Count the Number of R Waves: Count the number of R waves within this 6-second interval.

3. Calculate the Rate: Multiply the number of R waves by 10 to get the heart rate in bpm.

For example, if there are 7 R waves in a 6-second interval, the heart rate is:

$$7 \times 10 = 70\ bpm$$

The Sequence Method

The sequence method, also known as the "rule of 300," uses a sequence of numbers to estimate the heart rate quickly for regular rhythms.

1. Identify an R Wave on a Bold Line: Start with an R wave that falls on a bold line.

2. Apply the Sequence: Count the number of large boxes to the next R wave, applying the sequence: 300, 150, 100, 75, 60, 50.

For example, if the next R wave falls on the fourth large box after the starting R wave, the heart rate is approximately 75 bpm.

Heart Rate from Irregular Rhythms

For irregular rhythms, it's important to average the heart rate over a longer period to get a more accurate measure. The 6-second method is particularly useful here, but you can also use a longer interval, such as a 10-second strip (50 large boxes), and multiply the number of R waves by 6.

Practical Considerations

- Accuracy: For precise heart rate measurement, especially in critical care or research settings, use the 1500 method.

- Speed: For quick estimates in emergency or rapid assessment scenarios, the 300 method or sequence method can be handy.

- Irregular Rhythms: Always use the 6-second method or longer intervals for irregular rhythms to account for variability in the heart rate.

Determining heart rate from an ECG/EKG is a basic yet essential skill. The choice of method depends on the regularity of the rhythm and the need for accuracy versus speed. Understanding and practicing these methods will ensure accurate heart rate calculation in various clinical scenarios.

METHODS FOR CALCULATING RATE

Calculating heart rate from an ECG/EKG involves several methods, each tailored to different clinical scenarios or preferences:

1. Six-Second Method: Counting the number of QRS complexes in a 6-second strip and multiplying by 10 gives the heart rate per minute. This method is quick but less accurate for irregular rhythms.

2. 300 Rule: Dividing 300 by the number of large squares (0.2 seconds each) between consecutive R waves gives an approximate heart rate. This method is useful for regular rhythms.

3. 1500 Rule: Dividing 1500 by the number of small squares (0.04 seconds each) between consecutive R waves provides an approximate heart rate. This method is more precise for faster heart rates or when using faster paper speeds (e.g., 25 mm/s).

4. Counting R Waves: Counting the number of R waves in a full minute (or over a shorter duration and multiplying appropriately) provides an accurate heart rate.

5. Computerized Analysis: Modern ECG machines automatically calculate heart rate based on R-R intervals.

6. Calipers or Electronic Tools: Using calipers or electronic tools to measure R-R intervals on the ECG printout can provide precise heart rate calculations.

Each method has its advantages depending on the clinical situation, the patient's rhythm regularity, and the equipment available.

NORMAL, BRADYCARDIA, AND TACHYCARDIA

In ECG/EKG interpretation, understanding normal heart rate (HR), bradycardia, and tachycardia provides essential insights into the function and health of the cardiovascular system.

Here's a more detailed exploration:

Normal Heart Rate (HR)

A normal heart rate reflects the balance of electrical activity in the heart's conduction system, orchestrated by the SA node. The SA node generates electrical impulses that travel through the atria, causing them to contract and pump blood into the ventricles. The subsequent ventricular contraction completes the cardiac cycle, which is depicted as a regular and rhythmic pattern on the ECG/EKG.

On an ECG/EKG tracing of a normal heart rate:

- The R-R intervals (time between successive R waves) are consistent, indicating regularity in the heart's electrical impulses.

- P waves precede each QRS complex, representing atrial depolarization.

- QRS complexes are uniform and narrow, signifying rapid conduction through the ventricles.

A normal heart rate typically ranges between 60 to 100 bpm in adults. Factors influencing this range include age, fitness level, autonomic nervous system tone, and metabolic demands.

Bradycardia

Bradycardia refers to a heart rate that is slower than normal, typically below 60 bpm in adults. It can result from various physiological and pathological factors:

- Physiological Bradycardia: This can occur in well-trained athletes whose hearts efficiently pump blood with fewer beats per minute due to increased stroke volume and cardiac efficiency.

- Pathological Bradycardia: It may stem from abnormalities in the SA node, conduction system disorders (e.g., heart block), or side effects of medications (e.g., beta-blockers).

On an ECG/EKG tracing of bradycardia:

- The R-R intervals are prolonged, reflecting a slower heart rate.

- The P waves may appear normal if the bradycardia is due to sinus node dysfunction, or they may be abnormal if there is atrial conduction delay or block.

Clinically, significant bradycardia can reduce cardiac output and lead to symptoms such as dizziness, syncope (fainting), and fatigue. Management may involve identifying and treating the underlying cause, which could include pacemaker placement in severe cases.

Tachycardia

Tachycardia refers to a heart rate that is faster than normal, usually above 100 bpm in adults. It can be caused by physiological responses (e.g., exercise, stress) or pathological conditions:

- Physiological Tachycardia: During physical activity or emotional stress, the sympathetic nervous system increases heart rate to meet increased oxygen demands.

- Pathological Tachycardia: This can result from conditions such as arrhythmias (e.g., atrial fibrillation, ventricular tachycardia), fever, electrolyte imbalances, heart disease, or certain medications.

On an ECG/EKG tracing of tachycardia:

- The R-R intervals are shortened, indicating a rapid heart rate.

- Depending on the origin of tachycardia, QRS complexes may be narrow (supraventricular tachycardia) or wide (ventricular tachycardia).

Clinically, tachycardia can reduce cardiac filling time and impair cardiac output, leading to symptoms such as palpitations, shortness of breath, chest discomfort, and dizziness. Treatment depends on identifying and addressing the underlying cause, which may involve medications, cardioversion, ablation therapy, or other interventions.

Clinical Significance

Understanding normal heart rate variations and deviations like bradycardia and tachycardia is critical in clinical practice. These variations provide valuable diagnostic information about cardiac function and overall health. Regular monitoring and interpretation of ECG/EKG findings help healthcare providers assess cardiovascular status, guide treatment decisions, and improve patient outcomes.

ASSESSING HEART RHYTHM

Assessing heart rhythm in ECG/EKG involves a systematic evaluation of the regularity and characteristics of the electrical impulses generated by the heart. Here's a comprehensive explanation:

Heart rhythm assessment begins by identifying the presence and regularity of P waves and QRS complexes on the ECG/EKG tracing. The P wave represents atrial depolarization, while the QRS complex corresponds to ventricular depolarization. A normal sinus rhythm displays consistent P waves before each QRS complex, indicating regular atrial depolarization. Irregularities in this pattern may suggest arrhythmias.

Key steps in assessing heart rhythm include:

1. Rhythm Regularity: Determine if the R-R intervals (distance between successive R waves) are consistent throughout the tracing. Irregular intervals may indicate arrhythmias such as atrial fibrillation or atrial flutter.

2. P Wave Morphology: Assess the shape, duration, and amplitude of P waves. Normal P waves are smooth and upright in leads II and V1, suggesting sinus origin. Absent or abnormal P waves may indicate atrial enlargement or conduction abnormalities.

3. PR Interval: Measure the duration from the beginning of the P wave to the beginning of the QRS complex. Normal PR interval ranges from 0.12 to 0.20 seconds (3-5 small squares).

Prolonged PR intervals suggest atrioventricular (AV) conduction delay, seen in first-degree AV block.

4. QRS Complex: Evaluate the duration and morphology of the QRS complex. Normal QRS duration is ≤ 0.12 seconds (3 small squares) and typically appears as a narrow, upright waveform. Widened QRS complexes (> 0.12 seconds) may indicate bundle branch blocks or ventricular conduction delays.

5. ST Segment and T Wave: Examine the ST segment (period between QRS complex and T wave) and T wave morphology. ST segment elevation or depression may indicate myocardial ischemia or infarction. T wave abnormalities can signify electrolyte imbalances or myocardial injury.

6. Overall Interpretation: Integrate findings to classify the rhythm as sinus, atrial, junctional, or ventricular. Sinus rhythm is characterized by normal P waves preceding each QRS complex with a regular rhythm. Other rhythms may show absent P waves (as in junctional rhythms) or irregular patterns (as in atrial fibrillation).

7. Clinical Correlation: Consider clinical context and patient symptoms when interpreting rhythm findings. Symptoms such as palpitations, dizziness, or syncope may correlate with specific arrhythmias detected on the ECG/EKG.

By systematically evaluating these elements, healthcare providers can accurately diagnose arrhythmias, guide appropriate treatment, and monitor patient cardiac health effectively using ECG/EKG interpretations.

SINUS RHYTHM

Sinus rhythm is a term used in ECG/EKG interpretation to describe the normal electrical activity originating from the sinoatrial (SA) node of the heart.

Sinus rhythm is characterized by several key features on the ECG/EKG:

- Origin: The electrical impulse originates from the SA node, which is the natural pacemaker of the heart located in the right atrium.

- Rate: The normal sinus rhythm typically ranges between 60 to 100 beats per minute in adults, although it can vary slightly based on age and fitness level.

- Rhythm: The rhythm is regular, meaning the time interval between each heartbeat (RR interval) is consistent throughout the ECG tracing.

- P Wave: Each sinus beat is initiated by a P wave, which represents atrial depolarization (contraction). The P wave is typically upright in leads I, II, and aVF, and may be inverted in lead aVR.

- PR Interval: This interval represents the time it takes for the electrical impulse to travel from the SA node through the atria and reach the atrioventricular (AV) node. In sinus rhythm, the PR interval is typically between 0.12 to 0.20 seconds (3 to 5 small squares on ECG paper).

- QRS Complex: Following the PR interval, the QRS complex represents ventricular depolarization (contraction). It should be narrow (less than 0.12 seconds or 3 small squares), indicating that the impulse is conducted normally through the bundle branches and Purkinje fibers.

- QT Interval: This interval represents the total time for ventricular depolarization and repolarization. It should be within normal limits relative to the heart rate.

Sinus rhythm is considered normal and healthy, reflecting the heart's ability to generate and conduct electrical impulses effectively. Deviations from sinus rhythm may indicate various cardiac conditions or disturbances, such as arrhythmias originating from locations other than the SA node, or abnormalities in conduction pathways.

Sinus rhythm on an ECG/EKG is characterized by a regular rhythm, normal heart rate, and specific waveform characteristics (P wave, PR interval, QRS complex) that indicate normal electrical activity originating from the SA node of the heart.

ATRIAL RHYTHMS

Atrial rhythms in ECG/EKG refer to the patterns of electrical activity originating from the atria of the heart. These rhythms are crucial to understand as they can indicate various cardiac conditions and their implications for patient health.

Normal Sinus Rhythm (NSR)

Normal sinus rhythm is characterized by a regular, consistent pattern of electrical activity originating from the sinoatrial (SA) node. In NSR, the ECG shows:

- P waves that are upright and consistent in morphology.

- P waves precede each QRS complex.

- The PR interval is consistent and within normal limits (0.12 to 0.20 seconds).

- QRS complexes are of normal duration (0.06 to 0.10 seconds).

Atrial Fibrillation (AF)

Atrial fibrillation is a common arrhythmia characterized by chaotic electrical activity in the atria. In ECG:

- There are no distinct P waves; instead, there are rapid oscillations or fibrillatory waves.

- The ventricular response is irregularly irregular.

- QRS complexes are typically normal unless there is an underlying conduction abnormality.

Atrial Flutter

Atrial flutter is characterized by a rapid, regular atrial rhythm due to a re-entrant circuit within the atria. ECG findings include:

- Sawtooth-shaped flutter waves (F waves) between QRS complexes, typically in a 2:1, 3:1, or 4:1 ratio.

- Atrial rate is often around 250-350 beats per minute.

- Ventricular response may be regular or irregular depending on the conduction ratio.

Premature Atrial Contractions (PACs):

Premature atrial contractions are early depolarizations originating from ectopic foci within the atria. In ECG:

- Premature P waves may be different in morphology compared to sinus P waves.

- P waves occur earlier than expected, disrupting the normal sinus rhythm.

- The PR interval following the PAC may be normal or prolonged.

Understanding these atrial rhythms is essential for diagnosing and managing various cardiac conditions. Atrial fibrillation and atrial flutter, in particular, have significant implications for stroke risk and hemodynamic stability, requiring appropriate management strategies such as rate control, rhythm control, anticoagulation therapy, and, in some cases, cardioversion.

VENTRICULAR RHYTHMS

Ventricular rhythms on an ECG/EKG refer to abnormal heart rhythms that originate from the ventricles, the lower chambers of the heart. These rhythms are typically characterized by wide QRS complexes, as the electrical impulse spreads through the ventricles rather than through the normal conduction pathway of the atria and AV node.

Types of Ventricular Rhythms

- Premature Ventricular Contractions (PVCs): These are extra, abnormal heartbeats that begin in the ventricles. They are characterized by wide, bizarre-looking QRS complexes on the ECG. PVCs are common and can be benign, particularly in healthy individuals without structural heart disease.

- Ventricular Tachycardia (VT): VT is defined as three or more consecutive PVCs occurring at a rate of more than 100 beats per minute. It can be sustained (lasting longer than 30 seconds) or non-sustained (lasting less than 30 seconds). VT may cause symptoms such as palpitations, dizziness, or chest discomfort. Sustained VT can deteriorate into ventricular fibrillation.

- Ventricular Fibrillation (VF): VF is a life-threatening arrhythmia characterized by rapid, chaotic electrical activity in the ventricles. The ventricles quiver and are unable to pump blood effectively, leading to sudden cardiac arrest if not treated immediately with defibrillation.

Characteristics on ECG

- PVCs: Seen as premature QRS complexes that are wide (>0.12 seconds) and often bizarre in shape. They may not be preceded by a P wave, and the T wave following the PVC may be in the opposite direction of the QRS complex.

- VT: QRS complexes in VT are typically wide (>0.12 seconds) and may have a consistent morphology if monomorphic or varying morphologies if polymorphic. The rate is usually between 100 to 250 beats per minute.

- VF: On ECG, VF appears as rapid, irregular, and chaotic QRS complexes without discernible P waves or T waves. The rhythm is disorganized, and there is no effective cardiac output.

Causes and Clinical Implications

- Causes: Ventricular rhythms can result from various cardiac conditions such as myocardial infarction, cardiomyopathies, electrolyte disturbances (e.g., hypokalemia), and drug toxicity (e.g., certain antiarrhythmic drugs).

- Clinical Implications: PVCs are often benign in healthy individuals but may indicate underlying heart disease if frequent or symptomatic. VT and VF are more serious and require immediate intervention. VT can degenerate into VF, which is a medical emergency requiring prompt defibrillation to restore a normal rhythm and prevent sudden cardiac death.

Treatment

- PVCs: Treatment is generally focused on managing underlying causes such as electrolyte imbalances or reducing stimulants like caffeine.

- VT: Treatment may involve medications (e.g., antiarrhythmics), cardioversion, or catheter ablation for refractory cases.

- VF: Immediate defibrillation is essential. Advanced cardiac life support (ACLS) protocols are followed to manage VF, including CPR and medications such as epinephrine and amiodarone.

Understanding ventricular rhythms on ECG/EKG is crucial for healthcare providers to diagnose and manage potentially life-threatening arrhythmias effectively.

IRREGULAR RHYTHMS

Irregular rhythms in ECG/EKG refer to patterns of cardiac electrical activity that do not follow a consistent, predictable beat-to-beat interval. These irregularities can indicate various underlying cardiac conditions and may require careful analysis for accurate diagnosis and management.

One common irregular rhythm is atrial fibrillation (AF), characterized by chaotic and irregular electrical impulses originating from the atria. This results in an irregular ventricular response, often leading to an irregularly irregular rhythm on the ECG/EKG. AF is associated with increased risk of stroke due to ineffective atrial contractions and potential formation of blood clots in the atria.

Another irregular rhythm is atrial flutter, which manifests as a regular and rapid atrial depolarization at a rate typically around 250-350 beats per minute. This results in a characteristic "sawtooth" appearance of the atrial waves on the ECG/EKG. Atrial flutter can lead to symptoms similar to AF and also carries a risk of clot formation and stroke.

Ventricular arrhythmias, such as ventricular fibrillation (VF), are life-threatening irregular rhythms characterized by rapid and chaotic ventricular depolarizations. VF results in ineffective ventricular contractions and immediate loss of cardiac output, leading to cardiac arrest and requiring immediate defibrillation to restore normal rhythm.

Other irregular rhythms include various types of heart block, such as second-degree and third-degree atrioventricular (AV) block, which result in irregular conduction of electrical impulses between the atria and ventricles. These blocks can lead to symptoms ranging from mild dizziness to syncope and require careful monitoring and sometimes pacemaker insertion for management.

The interpretation of irregular rhythms on ECG/EKG involves careful assessment of the overall pattern, including the irregularity of R-R intervals (for irregularly irregular rhythms like AF), the presence of abnormal waveforms (such as fibrillatory waves in AF), and the relationship between atrial and ventricular activity. Treatment strategies depend on the specific rhythm disorder identified and may include medications, cardioversion, ablation therapy, or implantation of cardiac devices like pacemakers or defibrillators.

Understanding irregular rhythms is crucial for healthcare providers to promptly recognize and manage potentially life-threatening cardiac conditions, thereby improving patient outcomes and reducing the risk of complications such as stroke or sudden cardiac death.

CHAPTER 3

DIAGNOSING ARRHYTHMIAS

Diagnosing arrhythmias using ECG/EKG involves a systematic approach to analyzing the heart's electrical activity. An arrhythmia is any abnormality in the rate, regularity, or sequence of cardiac electrical impulses, which can manifest in various ways on an electrocardiogram (ECG/EKG).

When diagnosing arrhythmias, the ECG/EKG provides essential information about the heart's rhythm, rate, and the characteristics of each electrical waveform. Here's a comprehensive explanation of how arrhythmias are diagnosed using ECG/EKG:

Interpretation Process

1. Rate Assessment: The first step involves determining the heart rate by calculating the number of QRS complexes per minute. Normal heart rates range from 60 to 100 beats per minute (bpm) in adults.

2. Rhythm Analysis: After determining the rate, assess the regularity of the R-R intervals (or P-P intervals in atrial rhythms). Irregularities can indicate various types of arrhythmias, such as atrial fibrillation or multifocal atrial tachycardia.

3. Waveform Evaluation:

- P Waves: Assess the presence, morphology, and timing of P waves. Normal P waves precede each QRS complex, indicating normal atrial depolarization.
- QRS Complexes: Evaluate the duration (normal range 0.06-0.10 seconds) and morphology of QRS complexes. Wide QRS complexes (>0.12 seconds) can suggest ventricular arrhythmias or bundle branch blocks.
- ST Segment and T Waves: Analyze for elevation or depression, which may indicate myocardial ischemia, injury, or electrolyte disturbances.

4. Axis Determination: Determine the electrical axis of the heart to identify deviations that could suggest chamber enlargement or conduction abnormalities.

5. Additional Findings: Look for signs of conduction blocks (e.g., PR prolongation in AV blocks), presence of ectopic beats (e.g., premature atrial or ventricular contractions), or abnormal intervals (e.g., prolonged QT interval).

Clinical Correlation

Diagnosing arrhythmias using ECG/EKG requires correlating the findings with the patient's symptoms, medical history, and physical examination. It's crucial to differentiate benign arrhythmias from those requiring immediate intervention, such as ventricular tachycardia or severe bradyarrhythmias.

Reporting and Management

Once an arrhythmia is diagnosed, further investigations may be necessary to determine the underlying cause, such as echocardiography, stress testing, or Holter monitoring. Management strategies depend on the type and severity of the arrhythmia, ranging from observation to pharmacological intervention (e.g., antiarrhythmic drugs) or invasive procedures (e.g., catheter ablation or pacemaker implantation).

ECG/EKG interpretation is fundamental in diagnosing arrhythmias by assessing the heart's electrical activity, identifying abnormalities in rhythm and conduction, and guiding appropriate management strategies based on clinical findings.

ATRIAL ARRHYTHMIAS

Atrial arrhythmias are irregular heart rhythms originating from the atria, the upper chambers of the heart responsible for initiating the heart's electrical impulses. These arrhythmias are characterized by abnormal electrical activity in the atria, which can disrupt the normal sequence of heartbeats.

In an electrocardiogram (ECG/EKG), atrial arrhythmias often manifest as irregularities in the P-wave morphology and atrial activity. Common atrial arrhythmias include atrial fibrillation, atrial flutter, and atrial tachycardia. These arrhythmias can lead to ineffective atrial contractions and irregular ventricular rates, potentially compromising cardiac output and increasing the risk of thromboembolic events like strokes.

Atrial fibrillation (AF) is the most prevalent atrial arrhythmia, characterized by rapid and irregular atrial contractions without effective atrial systole. On an ECG/EKG, AF typically shows absent P waves and irregularly irregular R-R intervals. Atrial flutter, another common arrhythmia, presents with sawtooth-shaped flutter waves (F-waves) on the ECG and regular atrial rates. Atrial tachycardia, on the other hand, displays a rapid but regular atrial rate with normal P-wave morphology but may cause rapid ventricular response rates if not controlled.

Management of atrial arrhythmias involves identifying the underlying cause, controlling heart rate or restoring normal sinus rhythm, and preventing complications such as stroke through anticoagulation therapy in appropriate cases. Treatment strategies include medications to control heart rate (beta-blockers, calcium channel blockers) or rhythm (antiarrhythmic drugs), electrical cardioversion to restore sinus rhythm, and in some cases, catheter ablation to eliminate the arrhythmogenic focus.

Regular monitoring and management are essential due to the potential for these arrhythmias to worsen over time and their association with increased morbidity and mortality if left untreated.

PREMATURE ATRIAL CONTRACTIONS (PACS)

Premature Atrial Contractions (PACs) are a common type of cardiac arrhythmia seen on ECG/EKG tracings. They arise from the atria, the upper chambers of the heart, and are characterized by premature depolarizations of atrial tissue that occur before the next expected sinus beat

ECG/EKG Appearance of PACs

1. P Wave Characteristics:

   - PACs typically exhibit an abnormal P wave morphology compared to sinus beats.
   - The P wave may appear differently shaped, smaller, or with a different axis.
   - It may occur earlier than expected, occurring before the next expected sinus P wave.

2. R-R Interval:

- Following a PAC, there is usually a premature contraction of the atrium, resulting in a non-compensatory pause.
- The R-R interval after a PAC is shorter than the preceding R-R intervals.

3. Relation to Sinus Beats:

- PACs disrupt the normal sinus rhythm intermittently.
- They are often followed by a compensatory pause, where the subsequent sinus beat occurs slightly later to compensate for the early contraction caused by the PAC.

Clinical Significance

1. Symptoms:

- PACs are often asymptomatic but can cause palpitations or sensations of "skipped beats" in some individuals.
- Symptoms can vary depending on the frequency and timing of PACs.

2. Causes:

- Common causes include stress, fatigue, caffeine intake, and electrolyte imbalances.
- PACs can also occur in the setting of cardiac disease, such as atrial enlargement or ischemia.

3. Diagnosis and Differentiation:

- Diagnosis is made by identifying premature atrial depolarizations on ECG/EKG.

- It's important to differentiate PACs from other atrial arrhythmias like atrial fibrillation or atrial flutter, which have different ECG characteristics.

Management

1. Observation:

- Asymptomatic PACs often require no specific treatment.
- Monitoring may be necessary if symptoms are troubling or if PACs occur frequently.

2. Treatment of Underlying Causes:

- Addressing underlying factors such as stress reduction, caffeine limitation, and correcting electrolyte imbalances can help reduce PAC frequency.

3. Medical Intervention:

- In some cases, antiarrhythmic medications may be considered if PACs are frequent, symptomatic, or associated with underlying heart disease.
- Beta-blockers or calcium channel blockers may be prescribed to suppress ectopic atrial beats.

Prognosis

1. Generally Benign:

- PACs are typically benign and do not increase the risk of adverse cardiac events.
- However, frequent PACs or underlying heart disease may warrant closer monitoring and management.

2. Follow-Up:

- Regular follow-up with an electrophysiologist or cardiologist may be recommended, especially if PACs are symptomatic or associated with other cardiac issues.

Premature Atrial Contractions (PACs) are premature depolarizations originating from the atria, visible on ECG/EKG as abnormal P waves occurring earlier than expected. They are usually benign and often require no treatment unless symptomatic or associated with underlying heart disease. Recognition and differentiation from other arrhythmias are crucial for appropriate management and follow-up care.

ATRIAL FLUTTER

Atrial flutter is an abnormal heart rhythm characterized by rapid and regular atrial depolarizations (contractions) at a rate typically between 250-350 beats per minute (bpm).

ECG/EKG Characteristics of Atrial Flutter

1. Rhythm and Rate

- Rhythm: Atrial flutter presents as a regular, sawtooth pattern of atrial activity known as "flutter waves" or "F waves" on the ECG/EKG. These flutter waves have a characteristic appearance with a frequency of around 250-350 bpm.

- Rate: The ventricular response rate (ventricular rate) in atrial flutter depends on the conduction through the atrioventricular (AV) node. It can vary widely, often resulting in a 2:1, 3:1, or even 4:1 AV conduction ratio, meaning for every 2, 3, or 4 atrial beats, there is one ventricular beat respectively.

2. ECG Waveform Features:

- Flutter Waves: These are typically upright, uniform, and resemble the teeth of a saw on the ECG tracing. They appear between QRS complexes and are best seen in leads II, III, and aVF.

- QRS Complexes: Generally narrow (less than 0.12 seconds) if the conduction through the AV node is normal. Wide QRS complexes may indicate conduction abnormalities or underlying bundle branch block.

3. P Wave and PR Interval

- P Waves: Atrial flutter is characterized by the absence of discrete P waves. Instead, there are flutter waves that may be negative or positive, depending on lead orientation.

- PR Interval: The PR interval is not measurable in atrial flutter due to the absence of discrete P waves.

4. Atrial Rate and Atrial Activity

- The atrial rate in atrial flutter is extremely fast, typically between 250-350 bpm. This rapid atrial activity can lead to ineffective atrial contraction and contribute to symptoms such as palpitations and reduced cardiac output.

Clinical Significance and Symptoms

- Symptoms: Patients with atrial flutter may experience palpitations, dizziness, shortness of breath, and in severe cases, chest pain or syncope (fainting).

- Complications: If left untreated, atrial flutter can lead to more serious conditions such as atrial fibrillation, stroke (due to thromboembolism), and heart failure.

Management and Treatment

- Rate Control: Medications such as beta-blockers or calcium channel blockers are used to slow the ventricular response rate and improve symptoms.

- Rhythm Control: Antiarrhythmic drugs (like amiodarone, flecainide) or electrical cardioversion may be employed to restore normal sinus rhythm.

- Anticoagulation: Because atrial flutter increases the risk of blood clots forming in the heart, anticoagulant therapy (e.g., warfarin or direct oral anticoagulants) is often prescribed to reduce the risk of stroke.

Atrial flutter is a common arrhythmia characterized by rapid and regular atrial contractions seen as sawtooth-shaped flutter waves on ECG/EKG. Prompt diagnosis and appropriate management are crucial to alleviate symptoms, prevent complications, and improve patient outcomes. Understanding the distinctive ECG features of atrial flutter is essential for healthcare providers in diagnosing and managing this arrhythmia effectively.

ATRIAL FIBRILLATION

Atrial flutter is an abnormal heart rhythm characterized by rapid and regular atrial depolarizations (contractions) at a rate typically between 250-350 beats per minute (bpm).

ECG/EKG Characteristics of Atrial Flutter

1. Rhythm and Rate:

- Rhythm: Atrial flutter presents as a regular, sawtooth pattern of atrial activity known as "flutter waves" or "F waves" on the ECG/EKG. These flutter waves have a characteristic appearance with a frequency of around 250-350 bpm.

- Rate: The ventricular response rate (ventricular rate) in atrial flutter depends on the conduction through the atrioventricular (AV) node. It can vary widely, often resulting in a 2:1, 3:1, or even 4:1 AV conduction ratio, meaning for every 2, 3, or 4 atrial beats, there is one ventricular beat respectively.

2. ECG Waveform Features:

- Flutter Waves: These are typically upright, uniform, and resemble the teeth of a saw on the ECG tracing. They appear between QRS complexes and are best seen in leads II, III, and aVF.

- QRS Complexes: Generally narrow (less than 0.12 seconds) if the conduction through the AV node is normal. Wide QRS complexes may indicate conduction abnormalities or underlying bundle branch block.

3. P Wave and PR Interval:

- P Waves: Atrial flutter is characterized by the absence of discrete P waves. Instead, there are flutter waves that may be negative or positive, depending on lead orientation.

- PR Interval: The PR interval is not measurable in atrial flutter due to the absence of discrete P waves.

4. Atrial Rate and Atrial Activity:

- The atrial rate in atrial flutter is extremely fast, typically between 250-350 bpm. This rapid atrial activity can lead to ineffective atrial contraction and contribute to symptoms such as palpitations and reduced cardiac output.

Clinical Significance and Symptoms

- Symptoms: Patients with atrial flutter may experience palpitations, dizziness, shortness of breath, and in severe cases, chest pain or syncope (fainting).

- Complications: If left untreated, atrial flutter can lead to more serious conditions such as atrial fibrillation, stroke (due to thromboembolism), and heart failure.

Management and Treatment

- Rate Control: Medications such as beta-blockers or calcium channel blockers are used to slow the ventricular response rate and improve symptoms.

- Rhythm Control: Antiarrhythmic drugs (like amiodarone, flecainide) or electrical cardioversion may be employed to restore normal sinus rhythm.

- Anticoagulation: Because atrial flutter increases the risk of blood clots forming in the heart, anticoagulant therapy (e.g., warfarin or direct oral anticoagulants) is often prescribed to reduce the risk of stroke.

Atrial flutter is a common arrhythmia characterized by rapid and regular atrial contractions seen as sawtooth-shaped flutter waves on ECG/EKG. Prompt diagnosis and appropriate management are crucial to alleviate symptoms, prevent complications, and improve patient outcomes. Understanding the distinctive ECG features of atrial flutter is essential for healthcare providers in diagnosing and managing this arrhythmia effectively.

VENTRICULAR ARRHYTHMIAS

Ventricular arrhythmias are irregular heart rhythms originating from the ventricles, the lower chambers of the heart responsible for pumping blood to the lungs and the rest of the body. These arrhythmias can significantly impact cardiac function and are often visible on an electrocardiogram (ECG/EKG). Here's a comprehensive explanation focusing on ventricular arrhythmias:

Definition and Mechanism

Ventricular arrhythmias occur when the normal electrical impulses that coordinate heartbeats are disrupted, leading to abnormal rhythms originating from the ventricular myocardium. This disruption can cause the heart to beat too quickly (tachycardia), too slowly (bradycardia), or irregularly. The most common ventricular arrhythmias include ventricular tachycardia (VT) and ventricular fibrillation (VF).

Clinical Significance

These arrhythmias can impair the heart's ability to pump blood effectively, potentially leading to decreased cardiac output and compromised circulation. Ventricular arrhythmias are associated with conditions such as myocardial infarction (heart attack), structural heart disease, electrolyte imbalances, and adverse effects of medications.

Electrocardiographic Features

On an ECG/EKG, ventricular arrhythmias typically manifest as abnormal patterns in the QRS complex and T wave. Here are some key features:

- Ventricular Tachycardia (VT): Characterized by a series of three or more consecutive premature ventricular complexes (PVCs) occurring at a rate typically greater than 100 beats per minute. The QRS complexes are typically wide (>0.12 seconds) and bizarre in shape.

- Ventricular Fibrillation (VF): Represents a chaotic, disorganized electrical activity in the ventricles where there is no coordinated contraction of the heart muscle. On the ECG/EKG, VF appears as irregular, oscillating waves without identifiable QRS complexes or T waves.

Diagnostic Considerations

Diagnosing ventricular arrhythmias involves a thorough clinical assessment, including patient history, physical examination, and interpretation of ECG/EKG findings. Continuous monitoring with devices such as Holter monitors or event recorders may be necessary to capture intermittent arrhythmias.

Management and Treatment

Management of ventricular arrhythmias depends on the underlying cause, severity, and patient's clinical status.

Treatment strategies may include:

- Antiarrhythmic Medications: Drugs such as amiodarone, lidocaine, or beta-blockers may be used to stabilize the heart's electrical activity.

- Implantable Devices: Devices like implantable cardioverter-defibrillators (ICDs) can detect and terminate life-threatening arrhythmias such as VT or VF by delivering an electric shock.

- Catheter Ablation: In some cases, a catheter-based procedure may be performed to target and eliminate the source of abnormal electrical activity in the heart.

Prognosis

The prognosis for patients with ventricular arrhythmias varies depending on the underlying cause and the effectiveness of treatment. Early recognition, prompt intervention, and ongoing management are crucial in improving outcomes and reducing the risk of complications such as sudden cardiac arrest.

In summary, ventricular arrhythmias represent a diverse group of abnormal heart rhythms originating from the ventricles. Understanding their clinical significance, electrocardiographic features, and appropriate management is essential in providing optimal care for patients with these conditions.

PREMATURE VENTRICULAR CONTRACTIONS (PVCS)

Premature Ventricular Contractions (PVCs) are abnormal electrical impulses that originate from the ventricles of the heart and disrupt the normal rhythm established by the sinus node. Here's a comprehensive explanation about PVCs in the context of ECG/EKG interpretation:

Definition and Characteristics

Premature Ventricular Contractions (PVCs) are characterized by:

- Timing: They occur earlier than the next expected sinus beat.

- Appearance on ECG: PVCs appear as wide and bizarre QRS complexes, typically greater than 0.12 seconds (120 ms) in duration, due to abnormal depolarization originating from a ventricular focus.

- Compensatory Pause: After a PVC, there is usually a pause before the next sinus beat, as the sinus node resets its rhythm.

ECG/EKG Appearance

On an ECG/EKG strip, PVCs are identified by:

- QRS Complex: Wide (>0.12 sec) and bizarre in appearance.

- Absence of Preceding P Wave: Since the impulse originates from the ventricles, there is no preceding atrial depolarization (P wave).

- Compensatory Pause: Following the PVC, there is a pause before the next normal sinus beat, reflecting the refractory period of the ventricles.

Causes and Risk Factors

Common causes and risk factors for PVCs include:

- Structural Heart Disease: Such as coronary artery disease, myocardial infarction, cardiomyopathy, or valvular heart disease.

- Electrolyte Imbalance: Particularly hypokalemia (low potassium) and hypomagnesemia (low magnesium).

- Stress and Anxiety: Emotional stress or stimulant use.

- Caffeine, Nicotine, and Medications: Certain substances and medications can trigger PVCs.

- Age: PVCs are more common in older adults.

Clinical Significance

The significance of PVCs depends on:

- Frequency: Occasional PVCs are generally benign, but frequent or multiform PVCs can indicate underlying heart disease.

- Symptoms: Some individuals may experience palpitations, skipped beats, or discomfort.

- Complications: PVCs may contribute to decreased cardiac output if they occur frequently or in the context of structural heart disease.

Management and Treatment

Management of PVCs involves:

- Identifying and Treating Underlying Causes: Addressing electrolyte imbalances, reducing stress, and managing underlying heart conditions.

- Monitoring: Serial ECG/EKG monitoring to assess frequency and pattern of PVCs.

- Medications: In some cases, antiarrhythmic medications may be prescribed to suppress frequent PVCs.

- Lifestyle Modifications: Avoiding triggers such as caffeine, nicotine, and excessive alcohol. Managing stress through relaxation techniques or counseling.

Prognosis

- Benign vs. Malignant: PVCs are often benign in individuals without structural heart disease. However, in the presence of heart disease, they may indicate increased risk of arrhythmias or adverse cardiac events.

- Long-term Outlook: With appropriate management and treatment of underlying conditions, many individuals with PVCs have a good prognosis.

Premature Ventricular Contractions (PVCs) are abnormal heartbeats originating from the ventricles, characterized by wide QRS complexes on ECG/EKG. Understanding their appearance, causes, clinical significance, and management is crucial for accurate interpretation and patient care in clinical practice.

VENTRICULAR TACHYCARDIA

Ventricular Tachycardia (VT) is a potentially life-threatening arrhythmia characterized by rapid and regular firing of electrical impulses originating from the ventricles of the heart. In an ECG/EKG, VT typically appears as a series of wide QRS complexes (greater than 0.12 seconds) at a rate usually greater than 100 beats per minute (bpm).

ECG/EKG Characteristics of Ventricular Tachycardia:

1. QRS Complexes: Broad and bizarre in appearance, typically greater than 0.12 seconds in duration, due to abnormal ventricular depolarization.

2. Rate: Usually between 100-250 bpm, but can exceed this range.

3. Rhythm: Regular or slightly irregular.

4. P Waves: Typically absent or dissociated from QRS complexes. If visible, they may occur independently of the QRS complexes (atrioventricular dissociation).

5. ST Segment and T Wave: Often discordant with the QRS complexes, with ST segments and T waves usually in the opposite direction of the QRS complex.

Pathophysiology

Ventricular tachycardia arises due to abnormal electrical impulses originating from the ventricles, bypassing the normal conduction pathways.

This can occur due to various underlying conditions such as:

- Ischemic Heart Disease: Most commonly due to prior myocardial infarction (heart attack) leading to scar tissue.

- Cardiomyopathies: Structural heart diseases such as dilated cardiomyopathy or hypertrophic cardiomyopathy.

- Electrolyte Imbalances: Especially potassium and magnesium abnormalities.

- Drug Toxicity: Certain medications can predispose to VT by prolonging the QT interval or causing other electrophysiological disturbances.

Clinical Implications

- Hemodynamic Instability: VT can lead to decreased cardiac output and potentially progress to ventricular fibrillation, a more lethal arrhythmia.

- Symptoms: Patients may experience palpitations, dizziness, chest discomfort, or syncope (fainting).

- Complications: If sustained, VT can deteriorate into ventricular fibrillation, which can lead to sudden cardiac arrest if not promptly treated.

Management

1. Immediate Assessment: Confirm the rhythm and assess the patient's hemodynamic stability (pulse, blood pressure, consciousness).

2. Stable VT:

 - Administer antiarrhythmic medications such as amiodarone or lidocaine.

 - Consider synchronized cardioversion if medications are ineffective or if the patient becomes unstable.

3. Unstable VT (with signs of poor perfusion or hemodynamic compromise):

 - Immediate Cardioversion: Deliver a synchronized shock to terminate the arrhythmia and restore normal rhythm.

- Follow with antiarrhythmic medications to prevent recurrence.

4. Long-term Management:

- Address underlying causes such as ischemic heart disease or electrolyte imbalances.

- Consider implantable cardioverter-defibrillator (ICD) placement in patients at high risk for recurrent VT or sudden cardiac death.

Ventricular tachycardia is a serious arrhythmia that requires prompt recognition and intervention. ECG/EKG interpretation plays a crucial role in identifying and managing VT, aiming to restore normal cardiac rhythm and prevent potential life-threatening complications. Early diagnosis and appropriate management are essential in improving patient outcomes and reducing the risk of sudden cardiac death associated with this arrhythmia.

VENTRICULAR FIBRILLATION

Ventricular fibrillation (VF) is a life-threatening cardiac arrhythmia characterized by chaotic, rapid, and irregular electrical activity in the ventricles of the heart. This condition disrupts the heart's ability to effectively pump blood, leading to immediate loss of cardiac output and circulation. In an ECG/EKG, VF appears as a disorganized, irregular waveform without discernible P waves, QRS complexes, or T waves.

Pathophysiology of Ventricular Fibrillation

During VF, the normal coordinated contraction of the ventricles is replaced by rapid, uncoordinated electrical impulses originating from multiple foci within the ventricles. These impulses occur at a rate of 300 to 600 beats per minute, preventing the heart muscle from contracting effectively. As a result, blood flow to vital organs, including the brain and lungs, is severely compromised, leading to cardiac arrest and loss of consciousness within seconds if not treated promptly.

ECG/EKG Characteristics of Ventricular Fibrillation

1. Appearance on ECG/EKG:

- Absence of Normal Waveforms: VF is recognized by the absence of identifiable P waves, QRS complexes, and T waves. Instead, the ECG shows a rapid and irregular baseline with varying amplitudes and frequencies.

2. Irregular Rhythm: The ECG tracing in VF appears as a random, jagged line with no discernible pattern or regularity. This chaotic waveform contrasts sharply with the organized patterns seen in normal sinus rhythm or other arrhythmias.

Causes of Ventricular Fibrillation

VF often occurs in the setting of acute myocardial ischemia or infarction, where an area of the heart muscle becomes electrically unstable due to inadequate blood supply.

Other common causes include:

- Coronary artery disease (CAD): Blockage or narrowing of coronary arteries leading to reduced blood flow to the heart muscle.

- Electrolyte imbalances: Such as low potassium (hypokalemia) or low magnesium (hypomagnesemia).

- Cardiomyopathies: Structural abnormalities of the heart muscle that predispose to arrhythmias.

- Electrical shocks: From accidents or medical procedures that disrupt normal cardiac rhythm.

Clinical Implications and Management

Ventricular fibrillation is a medical emergency requiring immediate intervention to restore normal heart rhythm and circulation.

Effective management involves:

- Defibrillation: Prompt delivery of an electrical shock (defibrillation) to the heart is the most critical intervention. This shock aims to depolarize the entire myocardium simultaneously, allowing the heart's electrical system to reset and potentially restore normal sinus rhythm.

- CPR (Cardiopulmonary Resuscitation): If defibrillation is delayed or unavailable, high-quality CPR, including chest compressions and rescue breaths, can help maintain some blood flow to vital organs until advanced medical support arrives.

- Antiarrhythmic medications: Such as amiodarone or lidocaine may be administered to help stabilize the heart's electrical activity after initial defibrillation.

Prognosis

The prognosis of ventricular fibrillation depends heavily on the speed and effectiveness of treatment. Without immediate intervention, VF almost invariably leads to cardiac arrest and death. However, if treated promptly with defibrillation and advanced cardiac care, survival rates can be significantly improved, especially when coupled with timely CPR and access to emergency medical services.

Ventricular fibrillation represents a critical emergency in cardiology, characterized by rapid and chaotic electrical activity in the heart's ventricles. Early recognition through ECG/EKG findings, followed by immediate defibrillation and advanced cardiac life support measures, is crucial in restoring normal cardiac function and improving patient outcomes. Understanding the pathophysiology, ECG characteristics, causes, and management strategies for VF is essential for healthcare professionals involved in emergency and critical care settings.

JUNCTIONAL ARRHYTHMIAS

Junctional arrhythmias are abnormal heart rhythms that originate near the atrioventricular (AV) junction, where the atria and ventricles meet. These arrhythmias occur when the electrical signals in the heart deviate from their normal pattern. Typically, the sinoatrial (SA) node, located in the right atrium, generates the heart's electrical impulses, initiating each heartbeat. However, in junctional arrhythmias, the electrical signals may originate from within the AV node or the surrounding tissues.

In an ECG/EKG, junctional arrhythmias are characterized by specific changes in the P wave morphology. Instead of a typical P wave preceding the QRS complex, a junctional arrhythmia may present with a retrograde (inverted) P wave occurring either before, during, or after the QRS complex. The QRS complex itself usually appears normal in duration and morphology.

Clinically, junctional arrhythmias can manifest as different types of rhythms, such as junctional rhythm, accelerated junctional rhythm, or junctional tachycardia, depending on the heart rate and the origin of the electrical signals. These arrhythmias may occur due to various reasons, including dysfunction of the SA node, electrolyte imbalances, heart disease, or as a side effect of medications affecting cardiac conduction.

Management of junctional arrhythmias involves identifying and addressing the underlying cause. Treatment strategies may include pharmacological interventions to stabilize the heart rate and rhythm, correction of electrolyte abnormalities, or in severe cases, electrical cardioversion or placement of a pacemaker to regulate the heart's electrical activity.

Understanding junctional arrhythmias is crucial for healthcare professionals involved in interpreting ECG/EKG readings and managing patients with cardiac conditions, as prompt recognition and appropriate intervention can significantly impact patient outcomes and cardiac health.

JUNCTIONAL RHYTHM

Junctional rhythm is an important cardiac rhythm abnormality that can be identified on an electrocardiogram (ECG/EKG). It occurs when the electrical impulse of the heart originates from the atrioventricular (AV) junction rather than the sinoatrial (SA) node, which is the heart's natural pacemaker. Here's a comprehensive explanation of junctional rhythm:

Origin and Mechanism

The AV junction, also known as the atrioventricular node (AV node), is located near the tricuspid valve in the right atrium. Normally, the SA node initiates electrical impulses that travel through the atria, causing them to contract. These impulses then pass through the AV node to the ventricles, leading to their contraction.

In junctional rhythm, the SA node fails to initiate or conduct impulses properly. As a result, the AV junction takes over as the primary pacemaker of the heart. The AV junction has a slower inherent rate of electrical discharge compared to the SA node, typically ranging from 40 to 60 beats per minute (bpm).

ECG Characteristics

On an ECG, junctional rhythm is characterized by several key features:

- P Wave: The hallmark of junctional rhythm is the absence of a preceding P wave or a retrograde P wave that may appear just after the QRS complex. If present, the P wave may have an inverted shape (negative deflection) because it is generated in a retrograde fashion from the AV node towards the atria.

- QRS Complex: The QRS complex is typically normal in morphology and duration (less than 0.12 seconds), indicating normal ventricular depolarization.

- Rate: The heart rate in junctional rhythm depends on the location of the pacemaker within the AV junction. It ranges from 40 to 60 bpm in accelerated junctional rhythm and can exceed 60 bpm in junctional tachycardia.

- Rhythm: The rhythm appears regular if the AV junction consistently paces the heart at a regular interval.

Types of Junctional Rhythm

1. Normal Junctional Rhythm: Occurs when the AV junction naturally assumes the pacemaking role in the absence of SA node impulses. The rate is typically around 40 to 60 bpm.

2. Accelerated Junctional Rhythm: In this variant, the AV junction paces the heart at a rate of 60 to 100 bpm. It may occur transiently in response to physiological or pathological conditions, such as acute myocardial ischemia or digitalis toxicity.

3. Junctional Tachycardia: This is characterized by a rapid pacing rate of more than 100 bpm from the AV junction. It can be due to enhanced automaticity of the AV junction or triggered by sympathetic stimulation.

Clinical Significance

Junctional rhythms are generally considered benign when they occur transiently or in response to physiological stress. However, persistent junctional rhythms can indicate underlying cardiac pathology, such as atrioventricular node dysfunction, ischemic heart disease, or electrolyte imbalances (e.g., hyperkalemia). They may also be seen in patients recovering from cardiac surgery or those on medications affecting cardiac conduction.

Treatment Considerations

The management of junctional rhythm depends on its underlying cause and the patient's clinical status. Treatment strategies may include:

- Observation: Many cases of junctional rhythm are asymptomatic and transient, requiring only close monitoring.

- Correction of Underlying Causes: Addressing factors such as electrolyte disturbances, ischemia, or medication toxicity.

- Symptomatic Treatment: If the heart rate is excessively slow or fast and causing symptoms, interventions such as medications or temporary pacing may be considered.

In summary, junctional rhythm is an ECG finding where the AV junction becomes the primary pacemaker of the heart. Understanding its characteristics, types, and clinical implications is crucial for accurate diagnosis and appropriate management in clinical practice.

ACCELERATED JUNCTIONAL RHYTHM

Accelerated Junctional Rhythm is an electrocardiographic (ECG/EKG) finding that represents a rhythm originating from the atrioventricular (AV) junction at a rate faster than the typical junctional rhythm but slower than the normal sinus rate.

Definition and Origin

Accelerated Junctional Rhythm occurs when the automaticity of the AV junction increases, leading to the generation of electrical impulses at a rate typically between 60 to 100 beats per minute (bpm). This rhythm originates within the AV node or the junctional tissue near the AV node, which normally serves as a backup pacemaker in the absence of impulses from the sinus node.

ECG Characteristics

1. Rhythm: The rhythm is regular, meaning the distance between successive R-R intervals is consistent.

2. Rate: The heart rate typically ranges from 60 to 100 bpm. It is faster than the normal junctional rhythm (typically 40 to 60 bpm) but slower than the normal sinus rhythm (60 to 100 bpm).

3. P Wave: In Accelerated Junctional Rhythm, the P wave may be absent, retrograde (appearing inverted in relation to the QRS complex), or hidden within the QRS complex. This is because the impulse originates close to the AV junction, bypassing the atria or causing retrograde atrial depolarization.

4. QRS Complex: The QRS complex duration is typically normal (less than 0.12 seconds) unless there is an underlying conduction abnormality.

Causes

1. Enhanced Automaticity: Increased automaticity of the AV junction due to sympathetic stimulation, medications, electrolyte imbalances (e.g., hypercalcemia), or digitalis toxicity.

2. Atrioventricular Block: Accelerated Junctional Rhythm can occur as a compensatory mechanism in response to higher degrees of atrioventricular block (AV block), where impulses from the sinus node are not conducted effectively to the ventricles.

3. Pathological States: It may also be seen in pathological conditions such as myocardial ischemia, inflammation of the AV node (e.g., myocarditis), or following cardiac surgery.

Clinical Significance

Accelerated Junctional Rhythm itself may be benign and asymptomatic in many cases, especially when it occurs transiently. However, its presence can indicate underlying cardiac pathology or electrolyte disturbances that require further investigation and management.

Management

1. Observation: In asymptomatic patients with transient Accelerated Junctional Rhythm, observation may be sufficient without specific intervention.

2. Address Underlying Causes: Treatment focuses on correcting any reversible causes such as electrolyte imbalances, discontinuing offending medications, or managing ischemic heart disease if present.

3. Monitoring: Continuous ECG monitoring may be necessary in hospitalized patients or those with recurrent or symptomatic episodes to assess for changes in rhythm or potential complications.

Accelerated Junctional Rhythm is an ECG finding characterized by a regular rhythm originating from the AV junction at a rate faster than the normal junctional rhythm but slower than the sinus rate. It is important to understand its characteristics, causes, and clinical implications to provide appropriate management and further evaluation when necessary.

JUNCTIONAL TACHYCARDIA

Junctional tachycardia is an arrhythmia characterized by a rapid heart rate originating from the junctional tissue in the heart, specifically around the atrioventricular (AV) node. This type of tachycardia typically arises when the normal pacemaker of the heart (the sinoatrial or SA node) fails to maintain control over the heart rate, and the AV junctional tissue takes over as the primary pacemaker.

Mechanism and Causes

Junctional tachycardia can occur due to several reasons:

1. Enhanced Automaticity: Junctional tissue near the AV node may become irritable and spontaneously generate rapid electrical impulses, overriding the slower rate of the SA node.

2. Triggered Activity: Abnormal electrical impulses can be triggered within the junctional tissue, leading to rapid heart rates.

3. Reentry Mechanisms: In some cases, there may be a reentrant circuit around the AV node, where electrical impulses continuously circulate and stimulate the heart at a fast rate.

ECG/EKG Characteristics

When interpreting an ECG/EKG showing junctional tachycardia, the following characteristics are typically observed:

- Heart Rate: The heart rate is usually elevated, often between 100-150 beats per minute, but it can vary depending on the underlying cause and the individual's condition.

- Rhythm: The rhythm appears regular in most cases, but irregularities can occur depending on the specific origin and nature of the tachycardia.

- P Wave: Typically, P waves may be absent, retrograde (inverted before, during, or after the QRS complex), or buried within the QRS complex due to the junctional origin of the impulse. This occurs because the atria may not depolarize normally when the impulse originates close to the AV node.

- QRS Complex: The QRS complex is usually narrow (less than 0.12 seconds) unless there is an underlying bundle branch block or other conduction abnormality.

Clinical Significance and Management

Junctional tachycardia can present with symptoms ranging from palpitations, dizziness, and shortness of breath to more severe symptoms like chest pain and hemodynamic instability, depending on the rate and duration of the arrhythmia.

Management involves several approaches:

- Identifying Underlying Causes: Treatment depends on the underlying cause of the junctional tachycardia. It may be associated with electrolyte imbalances, cardiac ischemia, digitalis toxicity, or structural heart disease.

- Symptomatic Management: Initial management focuses on stabilizing the patient if symptoms are severe, using medications to control heart rate and potentially restoring normal rhythm through medications or electrical cardioversion.

- Long-Term Management: For recurrent or persistent junctional tachycardia, further evaluation and management by a cardiologist are necessary to determine if additional therapies such as catheter ablation or placement of a pacemaker are required.

Prognosis

The prognosis of junctional tachycardia depends on the underlying cause, the frequency of episodes, and the patient's overall cardiac health. With appropriate treatment and management, many patients can achieve good control of symptoms and maintain a good quality of life.

Junctional tachycardia is an arrhythmia characterized by a rapid heart rate originating near the AV node. Understanding its mechanisms, ECG/EKG characteristics, and appropriate management strategies are crucial for effectively diagnosing and treating this condition in clinical practice.

CHAPTER 4

CONDUCTION ABNORMALITIES

Conduction abnormalities in ECG/EKG refer to disruptions or delays in the electrical signals that control the rhythm and coordination of heartbeats. These abnormalities can be categorized into atrioventricular (AV) blocks and bundle branch blocks, each affecting different parts of the heart's conduction system.

Atrioventricular (AV) Blocks

AV blocks occur when there is an impairment in the transmission of electrical impulses from the atria (upper chambers of the heart) to the ventricles (lower chambers of the heart).

1. First-Degree AV Block:

- Description: Prolonged PR interval (>0.20 seconds).
- Cause: Often benign and asymptomatic; can be caused by medication effects or structural changes in the heart.
- ECG Characteristics: Every atrial impulse is conducted to the ventricles, but with delayed conduction through the AV node.

2. Second-Degree AV Block:

Type I (Wenckebach)

- Description: Progressive lengthening of the PR interval until a P wave is not conducted (dropped beat).
- Cause: Usually due to reversible conditions such as medication effects or ischemia.
- ECG Characteristics: PR interval prolongs until a beat is dropped, followed by a shorter PR interval.

Type II

- Description: Consistent PR interval with intermittently dropped beats (non-conducted P waves).
- Cause: Often due to structural heart disease affecting the His-Purkinje system.
- ECG Characteristics: PR interval remains constant, but occasionally a P wave is not followed by a QRS complex.

3. Third-Degree AV Block (Complete Heart Block):

- Description: No atrial impulses are conducted to the ventricles.
- Cause: Often due to severe structural heart disease or degenerative changes in the conduction system.
- ECG Characteristics: Atria and ventricles beat independently; P waves and QRS complexes are dissociated.

Bundle Branch Blocks

Bundle branch blocks occur when there is a delay or blockage in the electrical impulses traveling down the specialized pathways (bundle branches) that stimulate the ventricles to contract.

1. Right Bundle Branch Block (RBBB):

- Description: Delay in the electrical impulse through the right bundle branch.
- Cause: Often benign; can be seen in healthy individuals or due to pulmonary hypertension.
- ECG Characteristics: Widened QRS complex (>0.12 seconds) with an rSR′ pattern in V1 and V2.

2. Left Bundle Branch Block (LBBB):

- Description: Delay in the electrical impulse through the left bundle branch.
- Cause: Usually indicative of underlying heart disease such as coronary artery disease or cardiomyopathy.
- ECG Characteristics: Widened QRS complex (>0.12 seconds) with broad, notched or slurred R waves in V5-V6 and deep S waves in V1-V2.

Clinical Significance

Conduction abnormalities can vary in severity from benign conditions to potentially life-threatening situations. They are diagnosed primarily through ECG/EKG interpretation and clinical correlation. Management depends on the type and severity of the block, underlying conditions, and symptoms presented by the patient. Some may require close monitoring, adjustments in medications, or intervention with pacemakers to restore normal heart rhythm and prevent complications like syncope, heart failure, or sudden cardiac death.

Understanding these conduction abnormalities is crucial for healthcare providers to interpret ECG/EKG results accurately, make appropriate clinical decisions, and provide timely interventions when necessary.

ATRIOVENTRICULAR (AV) BLOCKS

Atrioventricular (AV) blocks are a group of conditions characterized by impaired conduction of electrical impulses from the atria to the ventricles through the AV node and the His-Purkinje system. These blocks can range from a mild delay in conduction to complete interruption of impulse transmission. Understanding AV blocks is crucial for the diagnosis and management of various cardiac conditions, as they can significantly affect heart function and patient outcomes.

Anatomy and Physiology of the AV Node

The AV node is a small structure located in the lower part of the right atrium near the septum. It serves as the electrical gateway between the atria and ventricles. The AV node slows down the electrical impulse, allowing the ventricles time to fill with blood from the atria before they contract. This delay is reflected in the PR interval on an ECG/EKG.

The AV node and the surrounding conduction system can be affected by various factors, including ischemia, medications, and intrinsic conduction system disease, leading to AV blocks.

Mechanism of AV Block

AV blocks occur due to a delay or complete interruption in the conduction of electrical impulses through the AV node or the His-Purkinje system. The severity of the block determines the clinical significance and the ECG/EKG findings.

ECG/EKG Features of AV Blocks

To identify an AV block on an ECG/EKG, it is essential to understand the normal components of the ECG/EKG tracing:

- P Wave: Represents atrial depolarization.

- PR Interval: Represents the time taken for the electrical impulse to travel from the atria through the AV node to the ventricles. The normal PR interval ranges from 0.12 to 0.20 seconds.

- QRS Complex: Represents ventricular depolarization.

General Characteristics of AV Blocks

AV blocks can be identified by analyzing the relationship between the P waves and the QRS complexes, as well as the duration of the PR interval.

Here are some general features to look for:

1. PR Interval Prolongation: A prolonged PR interval indicates a delay in conduction through the AV node. The normal range is up to 0.20 seconds.

2. Dropped Beats: In more advanced AV blocks, some P waves are not followed by QRS complexes, indicating that the atrial impulse did not conduct to the ventricles.

3. Regularity of P Waves and QRS Complexes: Assessing whether the P waves and QRS complexes occur at regular intervals can help determine the type of AV block.

Pathophysiology

AV blocks can result from various pathological processes, including:

- Ischemic Heart Disease: Ischemia can damage the conduction pathways, leading to AV block.

- Fibrosis and Degenerative Changes: Age-related changes can cause fibrosis of the conduction system, leading to block.

- Medications: Drugs such as beta-blockers, calcium channel blockers, and digoxin can slow conduction through the AV node.

- Inflammatory and Infiltrative Diseases: Conditions such as myocarditis, Lyme disease, and sarcoidosis can affect the AV node.

- Congenital Abnormalities: Congenital heart defects can involve the AV node and conduction system.

Clinical Significance

The clinical impact of an AV block depends on its severity:

- Mild Blocks (First-Degree): Often asymptomatic and found incidentally.

- Moderate to Severe Blocks (Second-Degree and Third-Degree): Can cause symptoms such as dizziness, syncope, and heart failure. Severe blocks may require urgent intervention.

Diagnosis

The diagnosis of AV block is primarily made using ECG/EKG. A detailed history and physical examination can provide clues to the underlying cause. Additional diagnostic tests, such as Holter monitoring, electrophysiological studies, and imaging, may be necessary to determine the etiology and guide treatment.

Management

The management of AV blocks depends on the type and severity of the block, as well as the underlying cause:

- Observation: Mild, asymptomatic blocks may require no treatment other than regular monitoring.

- Medication Adjustment: Discontinuing or adjusting medications that cause AV block.

- Pacemaker Implantation: Severe or symptomatic blocks often require the implantation of a pacemaker to maintain adequate heart rate and rhythm.

Atrioventricular (AV) blocks are important cardiac conditions that can significantly impact heart function and patient well-being. Recognizing the ECG/EKG features of AV blocks and understanding their pathophysiology, clinical significance, and management is crucial for healthcare providers in diagnosing and treating these conditions effectively.

FIRST-DEGREE AV BLOCK

First-degree atrioventricular (AV) block is a type of heart block in which the electrical conduction between the atria and ventricles of the heart is delayed but not completely interrupted. This delay occurs at the level of the AV node or the His-Purkinje system. In first-degree AV block, every atrial impulse is still conducted to the ventricles, but with a prolonged delay.

Electrocardiogram (ECG/EKG) Features

The hallmark of first-degree AV block on an ECG/EKG is a prolonged PR interval. The PR interval represents the time it takes for an electrical impulse to travel from the atria through the AV node to the ventricles. In first-degree AV block, the PR interval is consistently greater than 200 milliseconds (0.20 seconds) in duration.

Key ECG/EKG characteristics:

- PR Interval: Greater than 0.20 seconds (200 milliseconds).

- P Waves: Normal morphology and consistently followed by a QRS complex.

- QRS Complex: Normal duration and morphology, indicating that the delay is specifically in the AV node or His-Purkinje system and not in the ventricles.

Pathophysiology

First-degree AV block is typically caused by a delay in the conduction through the AV node or the His-Purkinje system. This delay can be due to a variety of factors, including:

- Enhanced Vagal Tone: Increased parasympathetic activity can slow down AV nodal conduction.

- Medications: Certain drugs can cause or exacerbate first-degree AV block, including beta-blockers, calcium channel blockers, digoxin, and some antiarrhythmic medications.

- Structural Heart Disease: Conditions that cause structural changes to the heart, such as ischemic heart disease, myocarditis, or cardiomyopathy, can affect AV nodal conduction.

- Electrolyte Imbalances: Abnormal levels of potassium, calcium, or magnesium can affect electrical conduction in the heart.

- Aging: Degenerative changes in the conduction system of the heart can lead to a first-degree AV block in older adults.

Clinical Significance

First-degree AV block is often asymptomatic and may be discovered incidentally during a routine ECG/EKG. In many cases, it does not require treatment or indicate a serious underlying condition. However, its presence may warrant further investigation to rule out other potential causes, especially if the patient has symptoms or if there is a known underlying heart condition.

Potential Symptoms:

- Usually Asymptomatic: Most individuals with first-degree AV block do not experience any symptoms.

- Rarely, Palpitations: Some may feel palpitations or an irregular heartbeat, though this is uncommon.

Management and Treatment

In most cases, first-degree AV block does not require specific treatment and can be monitored periodically. Management focuses on addressing any underlying conditions or contributing factors.

Treatment Strategies:

- Observation: Regular follow-up and monitoring, especially if the patient is asymptomatic and has no significant underlying heart disease.

- Adjusting Medications: If first-degree AV block is due to medication, adjusting the dosage or switching to an alternative drug may be considered.

- Addressing Underlying Conditions: Treating any underlying conditions, such as electrolyte imbalances or structural heart disease, can improve AV conduction.

Prognosis

The prognosis for individuals with first-degree AV block is generally good, particularly if there are no associated symptoms or underlying heart conditions. It is important for patients to have regular follow-ups to ensure that the AV block does not progress to a higher degree of block, such as second-degree or third-degree AV block, which could have more serious implications.

First-degree AV block is a condition characterized by a prolonged PR interval on the ECG/EKG. It is usually benign and asymptomatic, but it can be associated with certain medications, increased vagal tone, structural heart disease, and electrolyte imbalances. Management typically involves monitoring and addressing any underlying causes.

SECOND-DEGREE AV BLOCK (TYPE I AND II)

Second-degree AV block is a type of heart block where there is intermittent failure of atrial electrical impulses to reach the ventricles. This condition can be classified into two types: Mobitz Type I (Wenckebach) and Mobitz Type II. Below is a comprehensive explanation of both types without specifically delving into their distinct characteristics.

Second-degree AV block is characterized by the presence of some P waves that are not followed by QRS complexes. This implies that some impulses generated by the sinoatrial (SA) node do not successfully pass through the AV node to trigger ventricular depolarization. The clinical significance and treatment strategies differ between the two types of second-degree AV block, making it crucial to accurately identify and differentiate between them.

Pathophysiology

The primary issue in second-degree AV block is the intermittent failure of conduction from the atria to the ventricles. This failure can be due to various causes, including:

- Intrinsic AV Node Disease: Degenerative changes or fibrosis within the AV node can impair its function.

- Enhanced Vagal Tone: Increased parasympathetic activity can transiently slow down AV conduction.

- Myocardial Ischemia: Reduced blood flow, particularly affecting the AV node or His-Purkinje system, can lead to conduction disturbances.

- Medications: Certain drugs, such as beta-blockers, calcium channel blockers, and digoxin, can impair AV node conduction.

- Electrolyte Imbalances: Abnormal levels of potassium or magnesium can affect the electrical activity of the heart.

- Structural Heart Disease: Conditions like myocarditis, cardiomyopathy, or post-surgical changes can affect AV conduction.

Clinical Presentation

Patients with second-degree AV block may be asymptomatic or present with symptoms related to bradycardia and reduced cardiac output.

Common symptoms include:

- Palpitations

- Dizziness or lightheadedness

- Syncope or near-syncope

- Fatigue

- Shortness of breath

- Chest pain

The severity of symptoms often correlates with the degree of block and the presence of underlying heart disease.

Diagnosis

The diagnosis of second-degree AV block is primarily made using a 12-lead ECG. Key features on the ECG include:

- P Waves: Not all P waves are followed by QRS complexes. There will be intermittent non-conducted P waves.

- PR Interval: The PR interval can vary, particularly in Mobitz Type I, or remain constant in Mobitz Type II before the non-conducted P wave.

- QRS Complexes: The QRS complexes may be normal or widened, depending on the location of the block and any associated bundle branch block.

Management

The management of second-degree AV block depends on the type of block, the severity of symptoms, and the underlying cause. General approaches include:

- Observation: Asymptomatic patients or those with minimal symptoms, especially if the block is related to reversible factors, may be monitored without immediate intervention.

- Addressing Underlying Causes: Correcting electrolyte imbalances, adjusting medications that may contribute to AV block, and treating ischemia or other underlying conditions are essential steps.

- Pacemaker Implantation: Symptomatic patients, particularly those with Mobitz Type II block or those who experience significant bradycardia, syncope, or heart failure, may require a permanent pacemaker to ensure reliable ventricular conduction.

- Medications: In some cases, medications to increase heart rate and improve AV conduction may be used temporarily while awaiting further treatment.

Prognosis

The prognosis for second-degree AV block varies based on the type and underlying cause. Mobitz Type I generally has a more benign course and may not progress, especially if related to reversible causes. Mobitz Type II is more likely to progress to complete heart block and is associated with a higher risk of adverse outcomes, including syncope and sudden cardiac death, particularly if not treated with a pacemaker.

Second-degree AV block is an important condition to recognize and manage due to its potential impact on heart function and patient symptoms. Accurate identification through ECG, understanding the underlying pathophysiology, and appropriate management tailored to the patient's needs are essential components of care.

THIRD-DEGREE AV BLOCK

Third-degree AV block, also known as complete heart block, is a type of atrioventricular (AV) block where there is a complete disconnection between the atria and the ventricles. This means that none of the electrical impulses generated in the atria are conducted to the ventricles. As a result, the atria and ventricles beat independently of each other, each following its own intrinsic pacemaker.

Pathophysiology

In a healthy heart, electrical impulses generated by the sinoatrial (SA) node travel through the atria, causing them to contract, and then pass through the AV node to the ventricles, leading to coordinated contraction of the heart. In third-degree AV block, this pathway is completely disrupted at the AV node, bundle of His, or bundle branches.

The atria continue to follow the rhythm set by the SA node, typically at a normal rate (60-100 beats per minute), while the ventricles adopt a much slower rhythm, controlled by an escape pacemaker located either in the AV node, the bundle of His, or the Purkinje fibers. This ventricular rate is usually between 20-40 beats per minute if the pacemaker is in the bundle of His or Purkinje fibers, and slightly faster if the pacemaker is in the AV node.

ECG Characteristics

1. P Waves and QRS Complexes: There are P waves and QRS complexes present, but they occur independently of each other. There is no fixed relationship between the P waves and the QRS complexes.

2. Atrial Rate: The rate of the P waves (atrial rate) is typically faster than the ventricular rate.

3. Ventricular Rate: The rate of the QRS complexes (ventricular rate) is usually slow (typically 20-40 beats per minute).

4. P Wave Consistency: P waves are usually regular and consistent, but they can sometimes be hidden within QRS complexes or T waves.

5. QRS Duration: QRS complexes can be narrow or wide, depending on the location of the escape pacemaker. If the escape rhythm originates from the AV node or the bundle of His, the QRS complexes are usually narrow. If the escape rhythm is from the Purkinje fibers, the QRS complexes are typically wide.

Clinical Presentation

1. Symptoms: Patients with third-degree AV block often experience symptoms related to the slow ventricular rate and reduced cardiac output. These symptoms may include:

- Fatigue
- Dizziness or lightheadedness
- Syncope (fainting)
- Shortness of breath
- Chest pain
- Palpitations

2. Physical Examination: On physical examination, patients may have:

- Bradycardia (slow pulse)
- Hypotension
- Signs of heart failure (e.g., peripheral edema, jugular venous distention)

Causes

Third-degree AV block can result from a variety of conditions, including:

1. Ischemic Heart Disease: Myocardial infarction, especially involving the inferior wall, can damage the AV node or its surrounding tissues.

2. Degenerative Changes: Age-related fibrosis and sclerosis of the conduction system.

3. Cardiomyopathies: Diseases that affect the heart muscle, such as dilated cardiomyopathy or hypertrophic cardiomyopathy.

4. Inflammatory Conditions: Myocarditis, Lyme disease, or rheumatic fever.

5. Surgical or Procedural Complications: Cardiac surgery or catheter-based interventions that inadvertently damage the conduction system.

6. Medications: Drugs that can slow AV nodal conduction, such as beta-blockers, calcium channel blockers, or digitalis.

7. Congenital: Some patients are born with a congenital third-degree AV block.

Treatment

1. Temporary Measures: In an acute setting, temporary pacing may be necessary to maintain an adequate heart rate and cardiac output. This can be achieved using transcutaneous pacing (external) or transvenous pacing (internal).

2. Permanent Pacemaker: The definitive treatment for third-degree AV block is the implantation of a permanent pacemaker. This device ensures that the ventricles are paced at a rate sufficient to maintain adequate cardiac output and prevent symptoms. The type of pacemaker used typically involves dual-chamber pacing (DDD), which paces both the atria and ventricles and maintains AV synchrony.

3. Address Underlying Causes: Identifying and treating any reversible causes of the AV block is also important. This might include discontinuing or adjusting medications that affect AV nodal conduction, treating underlying ischemic heart disease, or managing infections or inflammatory conditions.

Prognosis

The prognosis of third-degree AV block largely depends on the underlying cause and the promptness of treatment. With appropriate pacing, patients can often return to a normal level of activity and have a good quality of life. However, untreated third-degree AV block can lead to severe complications, including heart failure, recurrent syncope, and sudden cardiac death.

BUNDLE BRANCH BLOCKS

Bundle Branch Blocks (BBBs) are abnormalities in the electrical conduction system of the heart, specifically within the bundle branches. The bundle branches are part of the heart's electrical wiring that transmits impulses from the atrioventricular (AV) node to the ventricles, leading to coordinated contractions. A block in one of these branches can delay or completely obstruct the electrical impulse, affecting the heart's rhythm and function.

Anatomy and Physiology of Bundle Branches

The heart's conduction system begins with the sinoatrial (SA) node, which generates an electrical impulse. This impulse travels through the atria to the AV node. From the AV node, the impulse moves into the His-Purkinje system, which includes the bundle of His, the right bundle branch, and the left bundle branch. The left bundle branch further divides into the left anterior and left posterior fascicles.

Pathophysiology of Bundle Branch Blocks

A Bundle Branch Block occurs when there is a disruption in the normal flow of electrical impulses through either the right or left bundle branch. This disruption can be due to various underlying conditions, such as ischemia, myocardial infarction, cardiomyopathy, or structural heart disease. When a block occurs, the affected ventricle receives the impulse later than the unaffected ventricle, causing a delay in contraction and an abnormal appearance on the ECG.

ECG Characteristics of Bundle Branch Blocks

The primary tool for diagnosing BBB is the electrocardiogram (ECG). Specific changes in the QRS complex, T wave, and ST segment help identify the presence of a block and its location.

General Features:

- Prolonged QRS Duration: Typically greater than 120 milliseconds.

- QRS Morphology: The shape of the QRS complex differs based on whether the block is in the right or left bundle branch.

Clinical Significance of Bundle Branch Blocks

The clinical significance of a BBB depends on several factors, including the presence of underlying heart disease, the type of block (right or left), and whether the block is complete or partial.

Symptoms:

- BBBs are often asymptomatic and found incidentally during an ECG.

- In some cases, patients may experience symptoms related to the underlying heart condition, such as syncope, palpitations, or heart failure symptoms.

Prognosis:

- Isolated Right Bundle Branch Block (RBBB) often has a benign prognosis, especially in the absence of other heart disease.

- Left Bundle Branch Block (LBBB) can be associated with a higher risk of adverse cardiovascular events, particularly if it occurs in the setting of ischemic heart disease or heart failure.

Management of Bundle Branch Blocks

The treatment of BBBs focuses on addressing the underlying cause. Specific management strategies include:

Monitoring:

- Regular follow-up and monitoring with ECG to assess for changes or progression.

Medications:

- Medications to manage underlying conditions, such as antihypertensives for hypertension or anti-ischemic drugs for coronary artery disease.

Interventional Procedures:

- Pacemaker implantation may be necessary for patients with symptomatic bradycardia or heart block.

- In cases of heart failure with reduced ejection fraction and LBBB, cardiac resynchronization therapy (CRT) may be beneficial.

Bundle Branch Blocks are conduction disturbances that impact the heart's ability to transmit electrical impulses effectively through the ventricles. While RBBB is often benign, LBBB can indicate more significant underlying heart disease and carries a different prognostic implication. Diagnosis is primarily made through ECG, and management focuses on treating the underlying conditions and monitoring for any progression of the block.

RIGHT BUNDLE BRANCH BLOCK (RBBB)

Right Bundle Branch Block (RBBB) is a cardiac conduction abnormality where there is a delay or blockage in the electrical impulses traveling through the right bundle branch of the heart's conduction system. This condition affects the right ventricle's ability to contract in a coordinated and timely manner. RBBB can be identified on an electrocardiogram (ECG/EKG) by specific patterns in the QRS complex.

Anatomy and Physiology

The heart's conduction system includes the sinoatrial (SA) node, atrioventricular (AV) node, bundle of His, and the left and right bundle branches. The right bundle branch conducts electrical impulses to the right ventricle. In RBBB, the conduction through this branch is delayed or completely blocked, causing the right ventricle to depolarize later than the left ventricle.

ECG/EKG Characteristics of RBBB

RBBB is diagnosed based on specific changes observed in the ECG/EKG:

1. QRS Complex Duration: Prolonged QRS duration greater than 120 milliseconds.

2. Lead V1 and V2 (Right Precordial Leads):

- rSR' pattern: The initial small r wave is followed by a deeper S wave and a secondary, taller R wave (R').
- Broad, slurred S waves.

3. Lead V5, V6, and Lead I (Left Lateral Leads):

- Wide S waves.

4. Secondary Repolarization Changes: Downsloping ST segments and inverted T waves in leads V1 and V2.

Causes of RBBB

RBBB can occur in individuals without any apparent heart disease or be associated with various cardiac and non-cardiac conditions:

1. Idiopathic: Often found in healthy individuals, particularly the elderly.

2. Structural Heart Disease:

- Ischemic heart disease (coronary artery disease)
- Cardiomyopathies
- Myocarditis

3. Pulmonary Conditions:

- Pulmonary embolism
- Chronic obstructive pulmonary disease (COPD)
- Pulmonary hypertension

4. Congenital Heart Disease:

- Atrial septal defect
- Tetralogy of Fallot

5. Trauma:

- Post-surgical (after open-heart surgery)
- Chest trauma

6. Electrolyte Imbalances: Severe hyperkalemia

Clinical Significance

The clinical implications of RBBB depend on the underlying cause:

1. Isolated RBBB: Often asymptomatic and found incidentally on ECG/EKG. It may not require any specific treatment if there is no underlying heart disease.

2. RBBB with Structural Heart Disease: Indicates the presence of more significant cardiac pathology and may be associated with an increased risk of adverse cardiac events. Further evaluation and management are necessary.

3. RBBB in Acute Settings: The presence of new-onset RBBB in the setting of an acute myocardial infarction or pulmonary embolism is a marker of severe disease and may necessitate urgent intervention.

Diagnosis

Diagnosis of RBBB is primarily made through an ECG/EKG. However, further diagnostic workup may include:

1. Echocardiography: To assess for structural heart disease.

2. Cardiac MRI: Detailed imaging of cardiac structure and function.

3. Stress Testing: To evaluate for ischemic heart disease.

4. Blood Tests: To identify underlying metabolic or electrolyte imbalances.

Management

Management of RBBB depends on the underlying cause and associated clinical conditions:

1. Asymptomatic RBBB: Typically, no treatment is required. Regular monitoring and follow-up are recommended.

2. Symptomatic RBBB or RBBB with Underlying Heart Disease:

- Treat the underlying condition (e.g., coronary artery disease, heart failure, pulmonary hypertension).
- In cases of symptomatic bradycardia or high-degree AV block, a pacemaker may be necessary.

3. Acute Management: In settings such as acute myocardial infarction or pulmonary embolism, treat the underlying acute condition urgently.

Prognosis

The prognosis of individuals with RBBB varies:

1. Isolated RBBB: Generally good, with minimal impact on overall mortality or morbidity.

2. RBBB with Underlying Cardiac Conditions: Prognosis depends on the severity and management of the underlying condition. RBBB can indicate an increased risk of cardiac events in these patients.

Right Bundle Branch Block is a conduction disorder characterized by delayed depolarization of the right ventricle.

While it can be benign in isolation, it may also be a marker of significant underlying heart disease. Proper diagnosis, evaluation, and management are crucial to address the potential implications of RBBB and associated conditions. Regular follow-up and monitoring are essential to ensure optimal patient outcomes.

LEFT BUNDLE BRANCH BLOCK (LBBB)

Left Bundle Branch Block (LBBB) is a condition that affects the conduction system of the heart, specifically involving the left bundle branch. To understand LBBB comprehensively, it's important to delve into its electrocardiographic (ECG) characteristics, clinical implications, underlying causes, differential diagnosis, management strategies, and prognosis.

Electrocardiographic (ECG) Characteristics of LBBB:

1. QRS Complex Widening:

- The defining feature of LBBB on ECG is a widened QRS complex, typically measuring greater than 120 milliseconds (ms) or 3 small squares on standard ECG paper. This prolonged QRS duration occurs because the left ventricle is depolarized via delayed activation after the right ventricle.

2. Specific QRS Morphology:

- Broad S Wave in Lateral Leads (I, aVL, V5, V6): These leads exhibit a broad, slurred initial downward deflection (S wave) due to delayed activation of the left ventricle.
- Broad R Wave in Right Precordial Leads (V1, V2): These leads typically show a broad, notched or slurred R

wave due to initial activation of the right ventricle followed by delayed left ventricular depolarization.

3. ST Segment and T Wave Changes:

- LBBB often causes secondary changes in the ST segment and T wave due to altered ventricular activation patterns. This includes ST segment depression and T wave inversion, particularly in leads with a predominantly negative QRS complex (e.g., V5, V6).

Clinical Implications

1. Diagnosis: LBBB is primarily diagnosed through ECG findings. It's essential to differentiate LBBB from other conditions that can mimic its ECG pattern, especially in the context of acute coronary syndromes.

2. Underlying Causes: LBBB can result from various underlying cardiac conditions:

- Ischemic Heart Disease: Such as myocardial infarction affecting the left bundle branch.
- Hypertensive Heart Disease: Chronic hypertension can lead to structural changes affecting the conduction system.
- Cardiomyopathies: Conditions like dilated cardiomyopathy can disrupt normal electrical conduction.
- Aging: Fibrotic changes associated with aging can affect the bundle branches.

Differential Diagnosis

- STEMI Mimicry: LBBB can mask the ECG changes typically seen in ST-elevation myocardial infarction (STEMI). Special criteria, like the Sgarbossa criteria, are used to identify acute myocardial infarction in the presence of LBBB.

- Other Conduction Abnormalities: Differentiating LBBB from other bundle branch blocks (e.g., right bundle branch block) and fascicular blocks is crucial for accurate diagnosis and management.

Management

- Treatment of Underlying Conditions: Management of LBBB focuses on treating the underlying cause, such as optimizing treatment for ischemic heart disease, hypertension, or cardiomyopathy.

- Monitoring: Regular follow-up with ECG and clinical assessment is necessary to monitor for progression or development of symptoms related to the underlying cardiac condition.

Prognosis

Varied Prognosis: The prognosis associated with LBBB depends on the underlying cause and the presence of associated cardiovascular conditions. It can range from benign to potentially life-threatening, especially if it signifies significant structural heart disease or increased risk of arrhythmias.

Clinical Considerations

Impact on Diagnosis: LBBB complicates the interpretation of ischemic changes on ECG due to altered QRS morphology. Clinicians must carefully evaluate clinical context and use additional diagnostic tools when necessary.

- Implications for Treatment: In some cases, LBBB may warrant specialized cardiovascular evaluation and treatment to manage associated risks, such as arrhythmias or heart failure.

Left Bundle Branch Block (LBBB) is a significant ECG finding that reflects disruption in the normal conduction pathways of the heart. Understanding its ECG characteristics, clinical implications, underlying causes, differential diagnosis, management strategies, and prognosis is crucial for effective clinical decision-making and patient care.

CHAPTER 5

ISCHEMIA AND INFARCTION

IIschemia and infarction are critical concepts in cardiovascular health, specifically concerning the blood supply to the heart muscle (myocardium).

Ischemia refers to a condition where there is reduced blood flow to a part of the myocardium. This reduction in blood flow can occur due to narrowing or blockage of the coronary arteries, which supply oxygen-rich blood to the heart muscle. Ischemia can be transient or chronic and may result from conditions like coronary artery disease (CAD), atherosclerosis, or vasospasm.

Infarction, on the other hand, occurs when ischemia is prolonged or severe enough to cause irreversible damage to the heart muscle. This irreversible damage results in tissue death (necrosis). Myocardial infarction (MI), commonly known as a heart attack, typically occurs when a coronary artery becomes completely blocked, usually by a blood clot (thrombus) that forms on top of a ruptured atherosclerotic plaque. The lack of blood flow leads to oxygen deprivation in the affected area of the heart, causing tissue necrosis.

Both ischemia and infarction can have serious implications for heart function and overall health. Prompt recognition and treatment are crucial in managing these conditions to minimize damage to the heart muscle and prevent complications such as heart failure or life-threatening arrhythmias.

Understanding the distinction between ischemia (reduced blood flow without tissue death) and infarction (tissue death due to prolonged ischemia) is essential for healthcare providers in diagnosing and managing cardiovascular diseases effectively. Treatment strategies aim to restore blood flow to the affected myocardium promptly, either through medications, procedures like angioplasty and stenting, or surgical interventions, depending on the severity and location of the blockage.

RECOGNIZING MYOCARDIAL ISCHEMIA

Recognizing myocardial ischemia on an ECG/EKG involves identifying subtle indicators that suggest inadequate blood flow to the heart muscle. While specific changes like ST depression or T wave inversion directly signify ischemia, understanding the concept behind these changes is crucial for accurate interpretation.

Myocardial ischemia occurs when there is insufficient blood supply to meet the oxygen demands of the heart muscle. This can result from atherosclerosis, coronary artery disease, or other conditions that limit blood flow through the coronary arteries. When ischemia occurs, the affected part of the heart muscle may not receive enough oxygen-rich blood, leading to biochemical and electrical changes that are detectable on an ECG/EKG.

During early stages of ischemia, the affected area may exhibit subtle changes on the ECG/EKG. These changes are often transient and may not be present continuously, making their recognition challenging yet vital. Clinicians look for deviations from the baseline pattern of the ECG/EKG, such as ST segment shifts, T wave alterations, or other morphological changes that indicate abnormal electrical activity.

Detecting myocardial ischemia on an ECG/EKG requires a systematic approach:

- Baseline Comparison: Understanding the patient's normal ECG/EKG pattern is essential. Deviations from this baseline may indicate ischemia.

- ST Segment Analysis: Typically, ischemia manifests as ST segment depression, indicating subendocardial ischemia, or ST segment elevation, indicating transmural ischemia.

- T Wave Changes: In some cases, T wave inversion can be an early sign of ischemia, particularly when associated with other changes.

Clinicians must consider patient symptoms, risk factors for cardiovascular disease, and the clinical context alongside ECG/EKG findings to accurately diagnose myocardial ischemia. Early recognition allows for prompt intervention, which is critical in minimizing myocardial damage and improving patient outcomes. Therefore, interpreting ECG/EKG changes indicative of ischemia requires both a keen understanding of cardiac physiology and a careful analysis of the ECG/EKG waveform.

ST DEPRESSION

ST depression on an ECG/EKG is a significant finding that often indicates myocardial ischemia, which refers to inadequate blood supply to the heart muscle. This condition can be caused by a variety of factors, including coronary artery disease (CAD), which is the most common cause, as well as other conditions affecting the heart's blood flow.

Characteristics of ST Depression

1. Appearance on ECG/EKG

    - ST depression is recognized as a downward deflection of the ST segment below the baseline, typically seen as a horizontal or downsloping depression.

- The depression is measured in millimeters and is significant when it exceeds 0.5 mm in the limb leads (I, II, III, aVL, aVF, and aVR) or 1 mm in the precordial leads (V1-V6).

2. Duration and Timing

- It can be transient (temporary) or persistent, depending on the underlying cause and the severity of ischemia.
- Transient ST depression may occur during stress testing or when the heart is under increased demand (e.g., during exercise or emotional stress).

3. Location

- The location of ST depression on the ECG can provide clues about the affected area of the heart.
- Typically, ST depression in leads V4-V6 suggests ischemia in the lateral wall of the left ventricle, while ST depression in leads II, III, and aVF may indicate inferior wall ischemia.

Interpretation and Clinical Significance:

1. Myocardial Ischemia

- ST depression reflects subendocardial ischemia, meaning that the inner layer of the heart muscle (myocardium) is not receiving enough oxygenated blood.
- It is an early sign of ischemia and may precede ST segment elevation in acute coronary syndromes (such as unstable angina or non-ST elevation myocardial infarction).

2. Differential Diagnosis

- Aside from CAD, other conditions can cause ST depression, including myocarditis, pericarditis, and ventricular hypertrophy.
- It can also occur due to electrolyte imbalances (e.g., hypokalemia), certain medications (e.g., digitalis), and physiological changes (e.g., during hyperventilation).

3. Clinical Management

- Prompt identification of ST depression is crucial for initiating appropriate management.
- Treatment focuses on addressing the underlying cause, such as optimizing coronary perfusion (e.g., with nitroglycerin or reperfusion therapy in acute coronary syndromes) and managing risk factors (e.g., hypertension, hyperlipidemia).

ST depression on an ECG/EKG is a vital clinical finding indicating myocardial ischemia. Its recognition and interpretation are pivotal in diagnosing and managing conditions affecting the heart's blood supply. Understanding the characteristics, location, and clinical implications of ST depression enable healthcare providers to make informed decisions regarding patient care and intervention strategies to prevent complications associated with ischemic heart disease.

T WAVE INVERSION

T wave inversion on an ECG/EKG refers to an abnormality where the normally positive deflection of the T wave becomes negative or inverted. This finding can be indicative of various cardiac and non-cardiac conditions, and its interpretation depends on clinical context, patient history, and accompanying ECG/EKG findings.

Causes of T Wave Inversion

1. Ischemia: One of the most common causes is myocardial ischemia, where insufficient blood flow to the heart muscle can lead to changes in the repolarization phase of the cardiac cycle. Ischemic T wave inversions are typically seen in leads facing the ischemic area.

2. Myocardial Infarction (MI): T wave inversion can occur after an acute myocardial infarction, particularly in the leads that correspond to the affected area of the heart. This inversion may persist for days to weeks post-MI.

3. Hypertrophy: Left ventricular hypertrophy (LVH) or right ventricular hypertrophy (RVH) can alter the normal pattern of repolarization, leading to T wave changes, including inversion.

4. Electrolyte Imbalance: Abnormal levels of potassium (hyperkalemia or hypokalemia) and calcium (hypercalcemia or hypocalcemia) can affect cardiac repolarization and manifest as T wave abnormalities.

5. CNS Disorders: Conditions affecting the central nervous system, such as intracranial hemorrhage or stroke, can sometimes cause T wave inversions on ECG/EKG.

6. Drug Effects: Certain medications, particularly those affecting cardiac repolarization (e.g., antiarrhythmics, psychotropic drugs), can induce T wave changes, including inversion.

7. Pericarditis: Inflammation of the pericardium can lead to diffuse T wave inversions, often accompanied by other ECG

changes such as PR segment depression and ST segment elevation.

Interpretation and Clinical Considerations

- Localization: T wave inversions can be localized or diffuse, depending on the underlying cause. Localized T wave inversions may point towards a specific coronary artery territory if due to ischemia or infarction.

- Chronic vs. Acute: Chronic T wave inversions may suggest longstanding myocardial changes, whereas acute inversions are more concerning for ongoing ischemia or recent myocardial injury.

- Clinical Correlation: Always interpret T wave inversions in conjunction with clinical symptoms, other ECG findings (e.g., ST segment changes), and patient history (e.g., cardiac risk factors, recent events).

- Dynamic Changes: T wave inversions that change dynamically with exercise or over time (e.g., during serial ECG monitoring) can provide valuable diagnostic information about the underlying condition.

T wave inversion on ECG/EKG is a significant finding that warrants careful evaluation and correlation with clinical context. It can indicate a range of cardiac and non-cardiac conditions, from ischemia and myocardial infarction to electrolyte disturbances and medication effects. Proper interpretation requires integrating ECG findings with patient history and clinical assessment to guide appropriate diagnosis and management.

IDENTIFYING MYOCARDIAL INFARCTION

Identifying myocardial infarction (MI) using ECG/EKG involves recognizing specific changes in the electrocardiogram that indicate ischemia or injury to the heart muscle. These changes are crucial for timely diagnosis and intervention.

Identifying Myocardial Ischemia on ECG/EKG

Myocardial ischemia refers to insufficient blood flow to the heart muscle due to partial or temporary blockage of coronary arteries.

ECG/EKG findings suggestive of myocardial ischemia include:

1. ST Segment Depression:

- Typically seen as a horizontal or downsloping depression of the ST segment from the baseline.
- Significant depression is defined as ≥0.5 mm (0.05 mV) in leads other than V1-V3, or ≥1.0 mm (0.1 mV) in leads V1-V3.
- The ST segment is measured from the end of the QRS complex to the beginning of the T wave.

2. T Wave Inversion:

- Inverted T waves can indicate myocardial ischemia, especially if they occur in conjunction with ST segment depression.
- T wave inversion is considered significant if it is ≥1 mm (0.1 mV) in depth and ≥0.04 seconds in duration.

3. Dynamic Changes:

- ECG/EKG changes with myocardial ischemia are often dynamic, meaning they may appear and disappear over time as ischemia fluctuates.
- Serial ECGs may be necessary to detect evolving changes indicative of ongoing ischemia.

4. Localization of Changes:

- The location of ST segment depression and T wave inversion can provide clues about the region of the heart affected by ischemia.
- For example, ST segment changes in anterior leads (V1-V4) suggest ischemia involving the anterior wall of the left ventricle.

Differential Diagnosis Considerations

When interpreting ECG/EKG changes, it's essential to consider other potential causes besides myocardial ischemia:

- Normal Variants: Certain individuals may have benign T wave inversions or ST segment changes that do not indicate ischemia.
- Electrolyte Imbalances: Abnormal levels of potassium, calcium, or magnesium can cause ECG/EKG changes similar to ischemia.
- Pericarditis: Inflammation of the pericardium can manifest as diffuse ST segment elevation with PR segment depression, mimicking myocardial infarction.

Clinical Correlation and Further Evaluation

- Clinical Presentation: ECG/EKG findings should always be interpreted in the context of the patient's symptoms, medical history, and clinical presentation.

- Serial ECGs: Changes over time (serial ECGs) can help confirm acute ischemia or infarction.

- Additional Testing: Confirmation of myocardial infarction typically requires cardiac enzyme tests (e.g., troponin levels) and possibly imaging studies (e.g., echocardiography, coronary angiography).

Identifying myocardial ischemia on ECG/EKG involves recognizing specific changes such as ST segment depression and T wave inversion. These findings, along with clinical correlation and further testing, help differentiate ischemic events from other causes of ECG/EKG abnormalities. Early recognition and intervention are crucial for improving outcomes in patients with acute coronary syndromes.

ST ELEVATION

ST elevation in an ECG (electrocardiogram) is a critical finding that indicates myocardial injury or infarction (heart attack). It is defined as an elevation of the ST segment above the baseline, typically seen in multiple contiguous leads. Understanding ST elevation is crucial for diagnosing and managing acute coronary syndromes.

Mechanism and Appearance

The ST segment on an ECG represents the interval between ventricular depolarization (completion of the QRS complex) and repolarization (onset of the T wave). Normally, the ST segment is isoelectric, meaning it is at the same level as the baseline.

ST elevation appears as a distinct upward deflection of the ST segment from the baseline. The elevation is measured in millimeters from the baseline to the point where the ST segment merges with the T wave. The morphology (shape) of the ST segment and any associated changes (e.g., T wave inversion, pathological Q waves) provide additional diagnostic clues.

Causes of ST Elevation

1. Acute Myocardial Infarction (AMI): The most common cause of ST elevation is acute transmural myocardial infarction, where there is complete occlusion of a coronary artery leading to ischemia and subsequent myocardial cell death. The affected leads typically correspond to the region of the myocardium supplied by the occluded artery (e.g., anterior wall infarction with ST elevation in leads V1-V4).

2. Pericarditis: Inflammation of the pericardium can cause diffuse ST elevation in multiple leads. The ST elevation in pericarditis is typically concave upwards (saddle-shaped), and there may be PR depression in leads opposite to where ST elevation is seen.

3. Early Repolarization: Seen as a benign finding in young, healthy individuals, early repolarization can sometimes mimic ST elevation myocardial infarction (STEMI). It is characterized by ST elevation with upward concavity and tall, peaked T waves.

4. Left Bundle Branch Block (LBBB): In the presence of LBBB, ST segment elevation can occur due to altered ventricular depolarization patterns. This can complicate the interpretation of ST elevation in these cases, requiring clinical correlation and sometimes additional imaging like echocardiography.

5. Brugada Syndrome: A genetic condition associated with abnormal sodium channels in the heart, leading to specific patterns of ST elevation in the right precordial leads (V1-V3) and an increased risk of sudden cardiac death.

Clinical Implications

ST elevation is a critical ECG finding that requires prompt evaluation and management:

- Diagnosis of STEMI: Immediate recognition of ST elevation myocardial infarction (STEMI) is crucial, as it mandates urgent reperfusion therapy (either through percutaneous coronary intervention [PCI] or thrombolytic therapy) to restore blood flow to the affected coronary artery and salvage myocardial tissue.

- Risk Stratification: The extent and magnitude of ST elevation, along with associated findings such as reciprocal changes and Q waves, help determine the size of the infarcted area and guide prognosis.

- Differential Diagnosis: While STEMI is a common cause, other conditions such as pericarditis, early repolarization, and even benign variants need to be considered based on clinical context, symptoms, and additional diagnostic tests.

ST elevation on an ECG is a crucial finding that necessitates urgent evaluation and appropriate management, especially in the context of acute coronary syndromes like STEMI. Understanding its causes, morphology, and associated findings is essential for accurate diagnosis and timely intervention to improve patient outcomes.

PATHOLOGICAL Q WAVES

Pathological Q waves on an ECG/EKG are significant indicators of myocardial infarction (MI) or other forms of myocardial injury.

Pathological Q waves are abnormal, deep, and wide Q waves that appear on an ECG/EKG. They are typically seen in specific leads and reflect significant myocardial tissue damage or necrosis. These Q waves are different from normal, small Q waves that can be seen in some leads of a healthy heart.

Causes

1. Myocardial Infarction (MI): The most common cause of pathological Q waves is a previous MI. During an MI, myocardial cells in the affected area become necrotic due to prolonged ischemia (lack of blood supply). This results in the loss of electrical activity and subsequent formation of deep Q waves on the ECG.

2. Myocardial Injury: Other forms of myocardial injury, such as myocarditis (inflammation of the heart muscle) or trauma to the heart, can also lead to pathological Q waves if they affect a significant portion of myocardial tissue.

Characteristics on ECG

- Depth and Width: Pathological Q waves are typically greater than one-third of the height of the R wave (or more than 0.04 seconds wide) in the same lead where they appear. They are often described as being deeper than normal Q waves and may have a sharp or wide appearance.

- Location: Pathological Q waves are usually seen in the leads that correspond to the area of the heart affected by the injury or infarction. For example, Q waves in leads V1-V4 indicate an anterior wall MI, while Q waves in leads II, III, and aVF indicate an inferior wall MI.

Clinical Significance

- Indicator of Myocardial Damage: Pathological Q waves are an important diagnostic marker for identifying previous myocardial damage. They help clinicians determine the location and extent of the infarction or injury, which guides further treatment and management decisions.

- Prognostic Value: The presence and characteristics of pathological Q waves can also provide prognostic information. Larger Q waves are associated with a greater extent of myocardial damage and may indicate a higher risk of complications or poor outcomes.

Differential Diagnosis

- Normal Variant Q Waves: In some cases, particularly in leads III and aVR, small Q waves may be normal variants and not indicative of pathology. It's important to differentiate between normal variants and pathological Q waves based on their characteristics and clinical context.

In summary, pathological Q waves on an ECG/EKG are abnormal deep and wide Q waves that indicate significant myocardial injury, most commonly due to myocardial infarction. They are crucial in diagnosing and assessing the extent of myocardial damage, guiding treatment decisions, and predicting patient outcomes. Prompt recognition and interpretation of pathological Q waves are essential skills in clinical cardiology and emergency medicine practice.

LOCALIZATION OF INFARCTION

Localization of infarction in ECG interpretation refers to identifying the specific region of the heart that has been affected by myocardial ischemia or infarction based on changes observed in the ECG/EKG. This localization is crucial as it helps clinicians determine the area of myocardium that has been deprived of oxygen and assess the potential extent of damage.

Key Concepts in Localization of Infarction

1. Electrode Placement and Leads:

- The 12-lead ECG records electrical activity from different perspectives or "leads" around the heart.
- Leads are categorized into limb leads (I, II, III, aVR, aVL, aVF) and precordial leads (V1 to V6), each providing a view from a specific angle relative to the heart.

2. Correspondence to Heart Anatomy:

- Each lead in the 12-lead ECG corresponds to a specific anatomical area of the heart.
- Leads V1 and V2 are positioned over the right ventricle and septum.
- Leads V3 and V4 are over the anterior surface of the left ventricle.
- Leads V5 and V6 are over the lateral wall of the left ventricle.
- Leads II, III, and aVF are oriented towards the inferior surface of the heart.

- Leads I, aVL, and aVR provide different views that assist in diagnosing specific conditions.

3. Recognizing Localization of Infarction:

- Anterior Wall: Infarction affecting the anterior wall of the left ventricle is typically identified by ST-segment elevation in leads V1 to V4.
- Inferior Wall: Infarction affecting the inferior wall, supplied by the right coronary artery (RCA), shows ST-segment elevation in leads II, III, and aVF.
- Lateral Wall: Infarction involving the lateral wall, often due to left circumflex artery (LCX) occlusion, presents with ST-segment elevation in leads I, aVL, V5, and V6.
- Right Ventricular (RV) MI: ST-segment elevation in lead V4R (right-sided V4) indicates RV involvement, commonly associated with proximal RCA occlusion.

4. Reciprocal Changes:

In infarction, reciprocal changes (ST-segment depression or T-wave inversion) in leads opposite the affected area may be observed, reflecting electrical vector changes due to myocardial injury.

5. Clinical Correlation:

Localization of infarction on ECG/EKG should always be correlated clinically with patient symptoms, history, and additional diagnostic tests (e.g., cardiac enzymes, echocardiography) to confirm the diagnosis and guide treatment.

Importance of Localization

- Treatment Planning: Helps guide urgent interventions such as thrombolytic therapy, percutaneous coronary intervention (PCI), or coronary artery bypass grafting (CABG).
- Prognostic Value: Differentiates between high-risk and lower-risk infarctions based on the extent and location of myocardial involvement.
- Long-Term Management: Guides decisions regarding medical therapy, rehabilitation, and risk factor modification to prevent future cardiovascular events.

By understanding the principles of localization in ECG/EKG interpretation, healthcare providers can promptly diagnose and manage acute myocardial infarction, improving patient outcomes and reducing morbidity and mortality associated with coronary artery disease.

ANTERIOR

Certainly! When referring to the anterior aspect in ECG/EKG interpretation, it typically relates to the leads that view the front of the heart, specifically leads V1 to V4 and sometimes extending to V5 and V6. Here's a comprehensive explanation:

Anterior Aspect in ECG/EKG Interpretation

The anterior aspect in ECG/EKG refers to the view of the heart's anterior wall from the perspective of specific leads on the ECG. This region includes the front of the heart, primarily encompassing the left ventricle and portions of the right ventricle.

Leads Involved

- V1 to V4: These are the primary leads that view the anterior aspect directly.

- V5 and V6: In some cases, these leads may also provide additional information about the anterior wall.

Characteristics and Interpretation

- P Wave: Represents atrial depolarization. Typically, it is upright in leads V1 to V3 and may be biphasic (positive/negative) or inverted in V4.

- QRS Complex: Reflects ventricular depolarization. In the anterior leads, a normal QRS complex should be narrow (less than 0.12 seconds in duration) and predominantly positive.

- ST Segment: Normally isoelectric (at baseline) in these leads. Deviations from baseline can indicate myocardial injury or ischemia.

- T Wave: Represents ventricular repolarization. It should be upright in leads V1 to V3 and may be positive or biphasic in V4 to V6.

Clinical Relevance

- Ischemia and Infarction: Changes in the ST segment and T wave in anterior leads (especially V1 to V4) can indicate myocardial ischemia or infarction affecting the anterior wall of the heart.

- Electrolyte Disturbances: Abnormalities in electrolytes like potassium or calcium can sometimes manifest with changes in the T wave morphology in anterior leads.

- Drug Effects: Certain medications can also alter the ECG pattern, particularly affecting the anterior leads due to their impact on cardiac repolarization.

Interpretive Tips

- Consistency in Lead Placement: Proper lead placement is crucial for accurate interpretation of the anterior aspect. Leads should be correctly positioned to ensure the heart's anterior wall is adequately captured.

- Comparison with Baseline: Always compare current ECG findings with previous recordings to identify any new or evolving changes, particularly in the anterior leads.

Understanding the anterior aspect in ECG/EKG interpretation helps clinicians assess cardiac health, identify abnormalities, and guide appropriate treatment strategies based on the observed patterns and changes.

INFERIOR

Inferior in the context of ECG/EKG refers to a specific region of the heart's electrical activity that is observed and analyzed through the leads placed on the lower part of the chest. This region predominantly involves the inferior wall of the left ventricle, which is supplied by the right coronary artery (RCA) and sometimes by the left circumflex artery (LCx).

ECG/EKG Leads Involved

The leads that primarily assess the inferior region include:

- II: The inferior limb lead, positioned on the lower left side of the chest.

- III: Another limb lead, which also provides information about the inferior aspect of the heart.

- aVF: The augmented vector foot lead, located on the lower right side of the chest.

Electrical Activity and Interpretation

Interpreting the inferior leads on an ECG/EKG involves several key observations:

1. P Wave: The P wave in these leads should normally be upright and consistent. Changes in the P wave morphology can indicate atrial abnormalities but are less specific for inferior myocardial infarction (MI).

2. QRS Complex: The QRS complex reflects the depolarization of the ventricles. In the inferior leads, a normal QRS complex should typically be narrow unless there are conduction abnormalities or bundle branch blocks.

3. ST Segment: This segment represents the early part of ventricular repolarization. In the inferior leads, the ST segment is particularly crucial for identifying myocardial ischemia or infarction. ST segment elevation (greater than 1 mm) in leads II, III, and aVF is highly indicative of acute inferior MI.

4. T Wave: The T wave represents ventricular repolarization. In normal conditions, it should be upright in leads II, III, and aVF. In the context of inferior MI, T wave inversion may occur during the recovery phase following ST segment elevation.

Clinical Significance

Identifying changes in the inferior leads is critical for diagnosing and managing conditions such as:

- Inferior Myocardial Infarction: ST segment elevation in the inferior leads is a hallmark of acute MI affecting the inferior wall of the heart.

- Ischemia: ST depression in these leads can indicate myocardial ischemia, suggesting inadequate blood supply to the inferior myocardium.

- Arrhythmias: Certain arrhythmias, such as atrioventricular blocks or junctional rhythms, may also manifest with characteristic changes in the inferior leads.

Differential Diagnosis

When interpreting an ECG/EKG, it's essential to consider differential diagnoses that could mimic or accompany the changes observed in the inferior leads. This includes considering patient history, symptoms, and additional ECG findings to differentiate between conditions like pericarditis, electrolyte disturbances, and non-cardiac causes of ST segment abnormalities.

In summary, understanding the significance of the inferior leads in ECG/EKG interpretation is crucial for promptly identifying cardiac conditions affecting the lower part of the heart. This knowledge enables healthcare providers to initiate appropriate interventions and optimize patient care based on the specific findings observed on the ECG/EKG.

LATERAL

In the context of ECG/EKG interpretation, "lateral" refers to a specific area of the heart that is being observed for abnormalities or changes in the electrical activity. The lateral wall of the heart is primarily represented by leads that are positioned on the left side of the chest and on the left arm.

Leads Involved in Lateral ECG Interpretation

The lateral leads typically include:

- V5 (placed on the left anterior axillary line, at the level of V4)
- V6 (placed on the left mid-axillary line, at the level of V5)
- I (the standard limb lead placed on the left arm)
- aVL (a modified limb lead also placed on the left arm)

Electrical Activity and Significance

The lateral leads on the ECG/EKG record the electrical activity of the left ventricle of the heart, specifically the lateral wall. Changes in the ECG/EKG in these leads can indicate various conditions affecting this area of the heart.

Common Findings in Lateral Leads

1. ST-Segment and T-Wave Changes

- ST-Segment Elevation: This may indicate myocardial infarction (heart attack) affecting the lateral wall of the left ventricle.

- T-Wave Inversions: Can suggest myocardial ischemia or myocardial injury, potentially indicating past myocardial infarction.

2. Axis Deviation

Deviations in the electrical axis of the heart seen in these leads may suggest underlying structural heart disease or changes in heart orientation due to physiological or pathological conditions.

3. Arrhythmias:

Certain arrhythmias, such as atrial fibrillation or ventricular ectopic beats, may manifest with characteristic changes in the lateral leads.

Clinical Interpretation

Interpreting ECG/EKG changes in the lateral leads requires a systematic approach, considering:

- Clinical History: Symptoms the patient presents with, such as chest pain or palpitations.
- Correlation with Other Leads: Comparing findings in the lateral leads with findings in other leads (e.g., anterior, inferior) to localize the area of concern.
- Serial ECGs: Comparing current findings with previous ECGs to assess for dynamic changes.

Understanding and interpreting the lateral leads in an ECG/EKG is crucial in diagnosing and managing cardiac conditions affecting the left ventricular lateral wall. It provides valuable information about the heart's electrical activity in that specific region, aiding in the diagnosis of myocardial ischemia, infarction, and other cardiac abnormalities.

POSTERIOR

Understanding the posterior leads in an ECG/EKG is crucial for a comprehensive assessment of cardiac electrical activity. Posterior leads are often referred to as the "right-sided ECG" or "posterior chest leads," and they provide additional information about the heart's electrical activity that is not fully captured by the standard frontal leads (I, II, III, aVR, aVL, aVF, V1-V6).

Anatomy of Posterior Leads

Posterior leads include:

- V7: Placed on the posterior axillary line at the level of V6.
- V8: Placed on the mid-scapular line at the level of V6.
- V9: Placed on the paraspinal line at the level of V6.

These leads are positioned on the back of the chest, providing a view of the heart's electrical activity from a different angle compared to the frontal leads.

Importance of Posterior Leads

1. Detection of Posterior Wall Myocardial Infarction (MI)

- Standard frontal leads may not adequately detect changes indicative of posterior wall MI due to the heart's orientation. Posterior leads are essential for identifying ST-segment depressions or elevations in the posterior wall, which are indicative of ischemia or infarction in these regions.

2. Enhanced Diagnostic Accuracy

- By incorporating posterior leads, clinicians can more accurately diagnose and localize myocardial ischemia or infarction. Posterior wall MI can present with ST-segment depressions in V7-V9, which may not be evident in standard leads.

Interpretation of Posterior Leads

- ST-Segment Changes: Look for ST-segment depressions or elevations in V7-V9. Ischemia or infarction affecting the posterior wall typically manifests as ST-segment depressions in these leads.

- Q Waves: Pathological Q waves in V7-V9 may indicate previous infarction or myocardial scar in the posterior wall.

- Integration with Frontal Leads: Interpret findings from posterior leads in conjunction with those from standard frontal leads to obtain a comprehensive assessment of the heart's electrical activity.

Clinical Application

Posterior leads are particularly useful in:

- Suspected Posterior MI: When clinical suspicion arises, especially if there are symptoms suggestive of ischemia (e.g., chest pain radiating to the back), posterior leads help confirm or rule out posterior wall involvement.

- Differentiating Etiology: Helps distinguish between anterior and posterior wall involvement in myocardial ischemia or infarction, guiding treatment decisions.

Posterior leads (V7-V9) provide critical additional information in ECG/EKG interpretation, particularly in detecting and localizing posterior wall myocardial infarction. Their integration into clinical practice enhances diagnostic accuracy and improves patient management by ensuring comprehensive assessment of cardiac electrical activity. Understanding and proficiency in interpreting posterior leads are essential for healthcare providers involved in cardiovascular care and ECG/EKG interpretation.

CHAPTER 6

ELECTROLYTE IMBALANCES AND DRUG EFFECTS

Electrolyte Abnormalities

Hyperkalemia

Hyperkalemia, characterized by elevated potassium levels in the blood, significantly impacts the heart's electrical activity and is readily observable on an ECG/EKG. Potassium plays a critical role in the cardiac action potential, and even slight increases can cause marked changes.

- Early Changes: One of the earliest signs of hyperkalemia is the appearance of peaked T waves. These T waves become tall, narrow, and symmetrical. This occurs because elevated potassium levels shorten the repolarization phase of the cardiac action potential.

- Progression: As hyperkalemia worsens, further changes become evident. The PR interval may prolong, indicating delayed atrioventricular (AV) conduction. The P waves can become flattened and eventually disappear, reflecting atrial paralysis.

- Severe Hyperkalemia: In severe cases, the QRS complex widens, leading to a sine wave pattern, which is a pre-terminal rhythm. This can quickly progress to ventricular fibrillation or asystole if not promptly treated. Immediate medical intervention, such as calcium gluconate administration to stabilize the cardiac membrane, and measures to lower potassium levels, are crucial.

Hypokalemia

Hypokalemia, or low potassium levels, also produces distinct ECG/EKG changes due to its effects on cardiac repolarization.

- Early Signs: One of the hallmark signs of hypokalemia is the flattening or inversion of T waves. Additionally, U waves, which are small deflections following the T wave, become more prominent. These changes are due to delayed repolarization.

- QT Prolongation: Severe hypokalemia can lead to a prolonged QT interval. This is particularly dangerous as it increases the risk of torsades de pointes, a specific type of polymorphic ventricular tachycardia that can degenerate into ventricular fibrillation.

- Arrhythmias: Besides torsades de pointes, hypokalemia can predispose patients to various arrhythmias, including premature ventricular contractions (PVCs) and atrial fibrillation.

Hypercalcemia

Hypercalcemia, or elevated calcium levels, affects the heart's electrical activity, primarily by shortening the QT interval.

- QT Shortening: The primary ECG/EKG manifestation of hypercalcemia is a shortened QT interval due to an abbreviated ST segment. This results from faster repolarization of the cardiac cells.

- Arrhythmias: While QT shortening is the most notable change, severe hypercalcemia can still increase the risk of arrhythmias, though less commonly than potassium imbalances.

Hypocalcemia

Hypocalcemia, characterized by low calcium levels, has opposite effects to hypercalcemia.

- QT Prolongation: Hypocalcemia leads to a prolonged QT interval due to a lengthened ST segment. This prolongation poses a significant risk for developing torsades de pointes.

- PR Interval: In addition to QT prolongation, hypocalcemia can cause a prolonged PR interval and, in severe cases, may lead to ventricular arrhythmias.

Drug Effects on ECG/EKG

Digitalis Effect

Digitalis glycosides, such as digoxin, are used to treat heart failure and certain atrial arrhythmias. They exert their effects by increasing intracellular calcium in cardiac cells, enhancing contractility, and reducing AV conduction.

- Characteristic Changes: The "digitalis effect" is characterized by a down-sloping ST segment depression with a "scooped" appearance, often referred to as the "digoxin effect." These changes are not indicative of myocardial ischemia but rather the therapeutic effect of the drug.

- Toxicity: At toxic levels, digitalis can cause a variety of arrhythmias. These include atrial tachycardia with block, junctional rhythms, and even life-threatening ventricular arrhythmias like ventricular tachycardia or fibrillation. Monitoring serum digoxin levels and electrolytes (particularly potassium) is essential in patients on digitalis.

Antiarrhythmic Drugs

Antiarrhythmic drugs are classified based on their primary mode of action on the cardiac ion channels.

- Class I (Sodium Channel Blockers): These drugs, such as quinidine, procainamide, and lidocaine, can widen the QRS complex and prolong the QT interval. They slow conduction velocity and can be used to treat various arrhythmias but must be used cautiously due to their proarrhythmic potential.

- Class II (Beta-Blockers): Beta-blockers, such as metoprolol and atenolol, slow the heart rate and prolong the PR interval by decreasing AV nodal conduction. They are effective for rate control in atrial fibrillation and for treating hypertension and ischemic heart disease.

- Class III (Potassium Channel Blockers): Drugs like amiodarone and sotalol prolong the QT interval by delaying repolarization. While effective in managing atrial and ventricular arrhythmias, they carry a risk of torsades de pointes.

- Class IV (Calcium Channel Blockers): These drugs, including verapamil and diltiazem, prolong the PR interval and can cause bradycardia by slowing AV nodal conduction. They are used to treat supraventricular tachycardias and for rate control in atrial fibrillation.

QT Prolongation

QT prolongation is a critical parameter to monitor as it can predispose patients to torsades de pointes, a potentially fatal arrhythmia.

- Medications: Several classes of drugs can prolong the QT interval, including antiarrhythmics (Class IA and III), certain antibiotics (e.g., macrolides, fluoroquinolones), antipsychotics (e.g., haloperidol, quetiapine), and antidepressants (e.g., tricyclics, SSRIs).

- Risk Factors: Patients with congenital long QT syndrome, electrolyte imbalances (especially hypokalemia and hypomagnesemia), and those on multiple QT-prolonging medications are at higher risk.

- Management: Monitoring the QT interval regularly in high-risk patients is crucial. If significant prolongation is detected, dose adjustment or discontinuation of the offending drug may be necessary, alongside correction of any electrolyte imbalances.

Understanding the ECG/EKG changes associated with electrolyte imbalances and various drugs is essential for clinicians. Recognizing these changes promptly can aid in diagnosing and managing the underlying conditions effectively, thereby preventing potentially life-threatening arrhythmias. Regular monitoring and a comprehensive approach to patient care, including electrolyte management and careful medication review, are vital components of safe and effective cardiac care.

ELECTROLYTE ABNORMALITIES

Electrolyte imbalances can significantly impact the electrical activity of the heart, often producing characteristic changes on an ECG/EKG. Understanding these changes is crucial for diagnosis and management. Below is a comprehensive explanation of the most common electrolyte abnormalities and their effects on the ECG/EKG.

Hyperkalemia

Hyperkalemia, an elevated level of potassium in the blood, affects the cardiac cells' resting membrane potential, leading to distinctive ECG/EKG changes. Early signs of hyperkalemia include peaked T waves, which are tall and narrow. As potassium levels increase, other changes can occur, including:

- Prolongation of the PR interval
- Widening of the QRS complex
- Loss of P waves
- Development of a sine wave pattern (a pre-terminal event)

Severe hyperkalemia can lead to life-threatening arrhythmias such as ventricular fibrillation or asystole.

Hypokalemia

Hypokalemia, a decreased level of potassium, can cause a variety of ECG/EKG changes due to its effect on myocardial repolarization. Typical findings include:

- Flattened or inverted T waves

- Presence of U waves, which are prominent, positive deflections following the T wave
- ST segment depression
- Prolongation of the QT interval

Severe hypokalemia can predispose patients to arrhythmias such as torsades de pointes, a specific type of polymorphic ventricular tachycardia.

Hypercalcemia

Hypercalcemia, an elevated level of calcium, shortens the duration of myocardial action potential, leading to characteristic ECG/EKG changes:

- Shortened QT interval, mainly due to a shortened ST segment
- In severe cases, Osborn waves (J waves) may appear, particularly at lower heart rates.

While hypercalcemia is less likely to cause arrhythmias compared to potassium imbalances, it can still lead to significant clinical symptoms and should be promptly addressed.

Hypocalcemia

Hypocalcemia, a decreased level of calcium, prolongs the repolarization phase of the cardiac cycle, resulting in:

- Prolongation of the QT interval, primarily due to lengthening of the ST segment

Prolonged QT interval in hypocalcemia increases the risk of developing torsades de pointes and other ventricular arrhythmias.

Magnesium Imbalances

Although not as commonly discussed as potassium and calcium, magnesium levels also play a critical role in cardiac electrophysiology.

- Hypermagnesemia (elevated magnesium levels) can lead to bradycardia, prolonged PR intervals, and widened QRS complexes. In extreme cases, it can cause heart block or asystole.
- Hypomagnesemia (low magnesium levels) is often associated with hypokalemia and can lead to prolonged QT intervals and an increased risk of torsades de pointes. It can also predispose patients to other ventricular arrhythmias.

Sodium Imbalances

Sodium imbalances generally have less direct impact on the ECG/EKG compared to potassium, calcium, and magnesium. However, severe hyponatremia (low sodium levels) can contribute to overall cardiac instability and predispose to arrhythmias, particularly in the presence of other electrolyte disturbances.

Clinical Management

Recognition and treatment of electrolyte abnormalities are crucial to prevent arrhythmias and other cardiac complications. Management typically involves correcting the underlying electrolyte imbalance:

- Hyperkalemia is treated with calcium gluconate for cardiac stabilization, insulin and glucose to shift potassium into cells, and potassium binders or diuretics to eliminate excess potassium.

- Hypokalemia requires potassium supplementation, either orally or intravenously, depending on severity.
- Hypercalcemia is managed with intravenous fluids, diuretics, and sometimes bisphosphonates to reduce calcium levels.
- Hypocalcemia treatment involves calcium supplementation, often intravenously for acute cases.
- Magnesium imbalances are corrected with magnesium supplements or cessation of magnesium intake, respectively.

Close monitoring with repeated ECGs/EKGs and laboratory tests is essential to ensure that electrolyte levels are corrected safely and effectively, minimizing the risk of arrhythmias and other complications.

HYPERKALEMIA

Hyperkalemia, an elevated level of potassium in the blood, significantly affects the electrical activity of the heart. Potassium is essential for maintaining the electrical membrane potential of cardiac cells, and any imbalance can lead to distinct and potentially dangerous changes in the ECG/EKG. Understanding these changes is crucial for timely diagnosis and effective treatment.

Early Signs of Hyperkalemia

In the early stages of hyperkalemia, when potassium levels are mildly elevated (5.5-6.5 mEq/L), the most noticeable ECG/EKG change is the presence of peaked T waves. These T waves are characterized by being tall, narrow, and symmetrical, often described as "tent-like." This occurs due to the increased rate of repolarization caused by elevated potassium levels, which makes the T waves sharper and more pronounced.

Moderate Hyperkalemia

As potassium levels rise to moderate levels (6.5-7.5 mEq/L), additional changes appear on the ECG/EKG. The PR interval, which represents the time between the onset of atrial depolarization and the onset of ventricular depolarization, begins to prolong. This prolongation is due to delayed atrioventricular (AV) conduction.

At this stage, the P waves, which represent atrial depolarization, may start to flatten or even disappear. This change reflects the increasing difficulty in initiating and propagating the electrical impulse through the atria. Concurrently, the QRS complex, which represents ventricular depolarization, begins to widen as the elevated potassium levels slow down the conduction through the ventricles.

Severe Hyperkalemia

In severe hyperkalemia (potassium levels above 7.5 mEq/L), the ECG/EKG changes become more pronounced and potentially life-threatening. The QRS complex continues to widen significantly, sometimes leading to a sine wave pattern. This pattern occurs as the QRS complex merges with the T wave, creating a smooth, undulating waveform that is a hallmark of severe hyperkalemia.

At this stage, P waves are often absent, indicating severe disruption in atrial electrical activity. The risk of developing serious ventricular arrhythmias, such as ventricular tachycardia or ventricular fibrillation, increases dramatically. These arrhythmias can quickly lead to cardiac arrest if not promptly treated.

Key ECG/EKG Features of Hyperkalemia

- Peaked T Waves: Tall, narrow, and symmetrical T waves are the earliest sign of hyperkalemia.

- Prolonged PR Interval: Reflects slowed atrioventricular conduction.

- Flattening or Disappearance of P Waves: Indicates severe atrial depolarization abnormalities.

- Widened QRS Complex: Shows slowed ventricular depolarization.

- Sine Wave Pattern: Fusion of the QRS complex and T wave in severe cases.

- Risk of Ventricular Arrhythmias: Includes ventricular tachycardia and fibrillation, which can lead to cardiac arrest.

Clinical Implications

Recognizing these ECG/EKG changes is critical because hyperkalemia can rapidly progress to life-threatening arrhythmias. Immediate treatment is necessary to lower potassium levels and stabilize the heart's electrical activity.

Management strategies include:

- Administration of Calcium Gluconate: This helps stabilize the cardiac membrane and counteract the effects of high potassium on the heart.

- Insulin with Glucose: Insulin helps drive potassium into cells, lowering extracellular potassium levels. Glucose is administered to prevent hypoglycemia caused by insulin.

- Sodium Bicarbonate: This can help shift potassium into cells, particularly in cases of acidosis.

- Diuretics: Medications that promote potassium excretion through the kidneys.

- Dialysis: Used in severe cases or when other treatments are ineffective, particularly in patients with renal failure.

Hyperkalemia manifests distinct, progressive changes on the ECG/EKG that correlate with the severity of potassium elevation. Early identification and prompt intervention are vital to prevent severe cardiac complications and ensure patient safety. Understanding these changes allows healthcare providers to respond effectively to this critical electrolyte disturbance, ensuring timely and appropriate management to mitigate the risks associated with hyperkalemia.

HYPOKALEMIA

Hypokalemia refers to a lower than normal level of potassium in the blood, typically defined as a serum potassium level below 3.5 mEq/L. Potassium is a crucial electrolyte involved in maintaining normal cell function, particularly in the heart. It plays a vital role in the electrical conductivity and muscle contraction of cardiac cells. When potassium levels fall below the normal range, it can lead to significant changes in the ECG/EKG, which can help in diagnosing and managing this electrolyte imbalance.

ECG/EKG Changes in Hypokalemia

The characteristic ECG/EKG changes associated with hypokalemia are due to its effects on the cardiac action potential. These changes include:

1. Flattened T Waves

One of the earliest and most common signs of hypokalemia on an ECG/EKG is the flattening or depression of T waves. T waves represent the repolarization of the ventricles. Low potassium levels delay this process, resulting in a less pronounced T wave. The amplitude of the T wave is reduced, and it may appear broader than normal.

2. ST Segment Depression

Hypokalemia can cause a downward displacement of the ST segment. This change is often subtle but can be observed as a slight downward slope from the baseline. The ST segment represents the period when the ventricles are depolarized and is normally isoelectric. In hypokalemia, the reduced extracellular potassium affects the resting membrane potential, leading to ST segment depression.

3. U Waves

The presence of prominent U waves is a hallmark of hypokalemia. U waves are small, positive deflections that follow the T wave. In hypokalemia, these waves become more noticeable and may even become larger than the T waves. U waves are thought to represent delayed repolarization of the Purkinje fibers. They are best seen in the precordial leads (V2 to V4) and can be mistaken for extra T waves.

4. Prolonged QT Interval

Hypokalemia can lead to a prolonged QT interval, which is the combined duration of the QRS complex, the ST segment, and the T wave. This prolongation increases the risk of developing dangerous arrhythmias, such as Torsades de Pointes. The QT interval prolongation is primarily due to the delayed repolarization of the ventricles, and it requires careful monitoring as it predisposes patients to potentially fatal arrhythmias.

5. ST-T Wave Changes

The overall morphology of the ST segment and T wave may show nonspecific changes, including subtle alterations in their shapes and slopes. The T waves may become biphasic or show flattening, and the ST segment may show a gentle downward slope.

Clinical Significance

The ECG/EKG changes seen in hypokalemia are important for several reasons:

1. Diagnostic Tool

The identification of these characteristic changes can prompt healthcare providers to measure serum potassium levels and confirm the diagnosis of hypokalemia. Early recognition on an

ECG/EKG can lead to timely intervention before the patient develops severe symptoms or complications.

2. Monitoring

Continuous ECG/EKG monitoring is essential in patients with hypokalemia, especially if they are at risk for severe complications. This allows for early detection of potentially life-threatening arrhythmias. Patients in intensive care units or those receiving treatments that affect potassium levels (e.g., diuretics) should have regular ECG/EKG monitoring.

3. Guiding Treatment

Recognizing ECG/EKG changes helps guide the treatment of hypokalemia, which typically involves potassium supplementation either orally or intravenously, depending on the severity. The ECG/EKG can be used to assess the effectiveness of the treatment and to ensure that potassium levels are being corrected safely.

4. Risk Stratification

Patients with prolonged QT intervals or prominent U waves may require more aggressive management and monitoring to prevent arrhythmias. Those with underlying cardiac conditions are at higher risk and need careful management to avoid adverse outcomes.

Causes and Risk Factors

Hypokalemia can result from a variety of conditions, including:

1. Increased Potassium Loss

- Diuretic Use: Loop and thiazide diuretics increase urinary potassium excretion.

- Gastrointestinal Losses: Vomiting, diarrhea, and nasogastric suction can lead to significant potassium loss.

- Renal Losses: Conditions such as hyperaldosteronism and renal tubular acidosis can increase renal potassium excretion.

2. Inadequate Potassium Intake

- Poor Dietary Intake: Insufficient dietary potassium can lead to hypokalemia, particularly in individuals with poor nutrition or restrictive diets.

- Total Parenteral Nutrition (TPN): TPN without adequate potassium supplementation can cause hypokalemia.

3. Shift of Potassium into Cells

- Alkalosis: Alkalosis causes potassium to shift from the extracellular to the intracellular space.

- Insulin Administration: Insulin promotes cellular uptake of potassium, reducing extracellular potassium levels.

- Beta-Adrenergic Stimulation: Beta-adrenergic agonists can drive potassium into cells.

Management

The management of hypokalemia involves:

1. Potassium Supplementation

- Oral Potassium Chloride: Commonly used for mild to moderate hypokalemia. It is available in various formulations, including tablets, capsules, and liquid.

- Intravenous Potassium: May be necessary for severe cases or when rapid correction is required. IV potassium must be administered carefully to avoid complications such as hyperkalemia and phlebitis.

2. Addressing Underlying Causes

- Identifying and treating the underlying cause of hypokalemia is essential to prevent recurrence. This may involve adjusting medications, treating gastrointestinal conditions, or managing hormonal imbalances.

3. Monitoring

- Regular monitoring of serum potassium levels and ECG/EKG is crucial during treatment to avoid hyperkalemia and ensure safe correction of potassium levels. Frequent checks are necessary in patients receiving IV potassium or those with significant ongoing potassium losses.

Complications of Untreated Hypokalemia

If left untreated, hypokalemia can lead to severe complications, including:

1. Cardiac Arrhythmias

- The most concerning complication is the development of potentially life-threatening arrhythmias, such as ventricular tachycardia, ventricular fibrillation, and Torsades de Pointes.

2. Muscle Weakness and Cramps

- Hypokalemia can cause generalized muscle weakness, cramps, and even paralysis in severe cases. This occurs because potassium is vital for normal muscle function.

3. Respiratory Distress

- Severe hypokalemia can affect respiratory muscles, leading to respiratory distress and failure. This is a medical emergency requiring prompt treatment.

4. Metabolic Alkalosis

- Hypokalemia can contribute to metabolic alkalosis, a condition where the blood becomes too alkaline. This occurs because potassium loss is often accompanied by hydrogen ion loss.

5. Rhabdomyolysis

- In rare cases, severe hypokalemia can lead to rhabdomyolysis, a condition where muscle tissue breaks down, releasing harmful substances into the bloodstream.

Hypokalemia has distinctive ECG/EKG manifestations that are critical for its diagnosis and management. Healthcare providers should be vigilant in recognizing these changes and understanding their clinical significance. Prompt and appropriate treatment can prevent complications and improve patient outcomes. Regular monitoring, both of potassium levels and ECG/EKG, is essential to manage this condition effectively and safely.

HYPERCALCEMIA

Hypercalcemia, an elevated level of calcium in the blood, can have significant effects on the electrical activity of the heart, which are reflected in characteristic changes on an ECG/EKG.

Pathophysiology

Calcium plays a critical role in cardiac muscle contraction and electrical conduction. Elevated calcium levels can shorten the duration of the action potential in cardiac cells by accelerating the inactivation of sodium channels and enhancing potassium efflux during repolarization. These changes impact the ECG/EKG readings in specific ways.

ECG/EKG changes in Hypercalcemia

Shortened QT Interval:

- The most notable ECG/EKG manifestation of hypercalcemia is a shortened QT interval. The QT interval represents the total time for ventricular depolarization and repolarization. Hypercalcemia accelerates ventricular repolarization, leading to a decreased duration of the QT interval.

- A shortened QT interval is due to the abbreviated ST segment rather than changes in the QRS duration or T wave.

Osborn Waves (J Waves):

- In severe hypercalcemia, you might see Osborn waves, also known as J waves. These are positive deflections occurring at the junction of the QRS complex and the ST segment.

- Osborn waves are more commonly associated with hypothermia but can be seen in hypercalcemia under certain circumstances.

Other ECG/EKG Findings:

- The PR interval and QRS complex typically remain normal in hypercalcemia.

- Although less common, hypercalcemia can lead to sinus bradycardia or other atrial arrhythmias due to its effects on the sinoatrial (SA) node and atrioventricular (AV) node conduction.

Clinical Significance

Identifying hypercalcemia on an ECG/EKG is crucial as it can be an indicator of underlying conditions such as primary hyperparathyroidism, malignancies (especially those with bone metastases), vitamin D toxicity, or excessive calcium supplementation. Recognizing the ECG/EKG changes can prompt further diagnostic testing and timely treatment, which is essential to prevent complications such as cardiac arrhythmias or sudden cardiac arrest.

Management

The treatment of hypercalcemia focuses on addressing the underlying cause and normalizing serum calcium levels. Acute management may involve:

- Intravenous Fluids: To promote renal excretion of calcium.

- Diuretics: Loop diuretics like furosemide may be used to increase calcium excretion.

- Bisphosphonates: These drugs inhibit bone resorption and are useful in malignancy-associated hypercalcemia.

- Calcitonin: This hormone helps to lower blood calcium levels rapidly.

- Dialysis: In severe cases, especially in those with renal failure, dialysis may be necessary to remove excess calcium from the blood.

Continuous monitoring of ECG/EKG is recommended during treatment to observe for resolution of the hypercalcemia-induced changes and to detect any potential arrhythmias that may arise during therapy.

Hypercalcemia has distinct ECG/EKG features, predominantly a shortened QT interval, which can aid in its diagnosis. Understanding these changes is vital for healthcare providers to manage and treat hypercalcemia effectively, preventing serious cardiac complications.

HYPOCALCEMIA

Hypocalcemia, characterized by abnormally low levels of calcium in the blood, can significantly influence the electrical activity of the heart, resulting in observable changes on an ECG/EKG. Calcium is a vital ion in cardiac physiology, playing an essential role in muscle contraction and the propagation of electrical impulses. Therefore, any disruption in calcium levels can have profound effects on cardiac function.

Mechanism of Hypocalcemia

Calcium ions are crucial for the contraction of cardiac muscle cells and the proper conduction of electrical signals in the heart. During the cardiac action potential, calcium enters the cells during the plateau phase (phase 2), facilitating the contraction of the heart muscle. In hypocalcemia, the reduced concentration of calcium ions affects this phase, altering the duration and characteristics of the action potential.

ECG/EKG changes in Hypocalcemia

The primary and most characteristic ECG/EKG change seen in hypocalcemia is the prolongation of the QT interval. This is mainly due to the lengthening of the ST segment, which reflects the phase of the action potential during which calcium ions enter the cardiac cells. Key ECG/EKG features of hypocalcemia include:

- Prolonged QT Interval: The QT interval represents the time from the beginning of ventricular depolarization to the end of ventricular repolarization. In hypocalcemia, the repolarization phase is extended, leading to a prolonged QT interval. This prolongation is a marker for an increased risk of arrhythmias, particularly torsades de pointes, a type of polymorphic ventricular tachycardia that can be life-threatening.

- Prolonged ST Segment: Specifically, the ST segment is lengthened in hypocalcemia. The ST segment represents the plateau phase of the cardiac action potential, during which calcium ions play a pivotal role. The prolongation of the ST segment is a distinguishing feature of hypocalcemia and helps differentiate it from other causes of QT prolongation.

Clinical Implications

The prolongation of the QT interval due to hypocalcemia increases the risk of serious arrhythmias. Torsades de pointes is of particular concern because it can degenerate into ventricular fibrillation, leading to sudden cardiac arrest if not promptly treated. Therefore, it is crucial to identify and correct hypocalcemia early to prevent such complications.

Management of Hypocalcemia

Management involves addressing the underlying cause of hypocalcemia and restoring normal calcium levels. This typically involves:

- Calcium Supplementation: Calcium can be administered orally for mild hypocalcemia or intravenously for severe cases. Intravenous calcium is often given as calcium gluconate or calcium chloride, depending on the clinical situation.

- Monitoring and Follow-Up: Continuous ECG/EKG monitoring may be necessary for patients with severe hypocalcemia or those receiving intravenous calcium to quickly detect and manage any arrhythmias. Blood calcium levels should be regularly monitored to ensure they return to and remain within the normal range.

Diagnosis and Monitoring

The diagnosis of hypocalcemia is confirmed through blood tests showing low serum calcium levels. It is essential to perform an ECG/EKG once hypocalcemia is suspected or diagnosed to detect any changes and assess the risk of arrhythmias. ECG/EKG findings, coupled with clinical symptoms such as muscle cramps, tetany, or seizures, can help guide the diagnosis and treatment plan.

Hypocalcemia can significantly impact cardiac function and manifest on an ECG/EKG primarily through the prolongation of the QT interval and the ST segment. Recognizing these changes is crucial for early diagnosis and prompt treatment, thus preventing the development of potentially life-threatening arrhythmias. Regular monitoring of ECG/EKG and serum calcium levels, along with appropriate management, is vital to ensure patient safety and optimal cardiac health.

DRUG EFFECTS ON ECG/EKG

Drugs can significantly impact the heart's electrical activity, and these effects are often reflected on an ECG/EKG. Understanding these changes is crucial for clinicians to accurately interpret ECGs and manage patients on various medications.

Antiarrhythmic Drugs

Antiarrhythmic drugs are designed to treat abnormal heart rhythms. They can have complex effects on the ECG, depending on the specific class of the drug.

1. Class I (Sodium Channel Blockers): These drugs, such as quinidine, procainamide, and lidocaine, primarily affect the QRS complex by slowing conduction through the heart's electrical system. This can cause a widening of the QRS complex. They are subdivided into three groups:

- Class IA: Quinidine, procainamide, and disopyramide prolong the action potential duration and refractory period, leading to a prolonged QT interval.
- Class IB: Lidocaine and mexiletine shorten the action potential duration, primarily used for ventricular arrhythmias and often have minimal effect on the ECG at therapeutic doses.
- Class IC: Flecainide and propafenone significantly slow conduction without much effect on the action potential duration, leading to a marked widening of the QRS complex.

2. Class II (Beta Blockers): Drugs like metoprolol, atenolol, and propranolol decrease heart rate and reduce the force of contraction by inhibiting sympathetic activity. On the ECG, beta blockers primarily cause a reduction in the heart rate (bradycardia) and may prolong the PR interval due to slowed conduction through the AV node.

3. Class III (Potassium Channel Blockers): Amiodarone, sotalol, dofetilide, and ibutilide prolong repolarization, reflected as a prolonged QT interval on the ECG. This can increase the risk of torsades de pointes, a potentially life-threatening arrhythmia. Amiodarone has complex effects, also exhibiting some properties of other antiarrhythmic classes, leading to a potential increase in QRS duration and PR interval.

4. Class IV (Calcium Channel Blockers): Verapamil and diltiazem slow the conduction through the AV node, leading to a prolonged PR interval and a slower heart rate. They are primarily used for controlling heart rate in supraventricular tachycardias.

Digitalis (Digoxin)

Digoxin is used to treat atrial fibrillation and heart failure. It has distinct effects on the ECG, known as the "digoxin effect," which includes:

- A scooped ST segment depression (often described as a "hockey stick" or "reverse tick" appearance).

- A shortened QT interval due to accelerated repolarization.

- An increased PR interval due to slowed conduction through the AV node.

- Potential arrhythmias, including premature ventricular contractions (PVCs), atrial tachycardia with block, and bidirectional ventricular tachycardia. These arrhythmias can be exacerbated by electrolyte imbalances, especially hypokalemia, which enhances digoxin's effects.

QT-Prolonging Drugs

Many drugs can prolong the QT interval, increasing the risk of torsades de pointes, a specific type of polymorphic ventricular tachycardia. These drugs include:

- Antibiotics: Macrolides (e.g., erythromycin, clarithromycin) and fluoroquinolones (e.g., levofloxacin, ciprofloxacin) can prolong the QT interval.

- Antipsychotics: Drugs like haloperidol, quetiapine, and ziprasidone can cause QT prolongation.

- Antidepressants: Tricyclic antidepressants (e.g., amitriptyline) and selective serotonin reuptake inhibitors (SSRIs) like citalopram can prolong the QT interval.

- Antiarrhythmics: As mentioned earlier, Class IA and Class III antiarrhythmics are significant contributors to QT prolongation.

- Other drugs: Some antihistamines (e.g., diphenhydramine in high doses), antifungals (e.g., fluconazole), and methadone.

Monitoring the QT interval is essential when patients are on these medications, especially when combining multiple QT-prolonging drugs or in the presence of other risk factors such as electrolyte imbalances.

Other Drug Effects

- Diuretics: These drugs, especially loop (e.g., furosemide) and thiazide diuretics (e.g., hydrochlorothiazide), can cause electrolyte imbalances such as hypokalemia and hypomagnesemia, which in turn can lead to ECG changes. Hypokalemia can cause:

  - Flattened or inverted T waves.

  - The appearance of U waves.

  - ST depression.

  Severe hypokalemia can lead to prolonged QT intervals and increase the risk of arrhythmias.

- Lithium: Used in psychiatric disorders, lithium can cause T wave flattening or inversion, and at toxic levels, it can lead to various arrhythmias, including sinus node dysfunction and AV block.

- Tricyclic Antidepressants (TCAs): Overdose of TCAs can cause sinus tachycardia, prolonged PR, QRS, and QT intervals, and may lead to life-threatening arrhythmias such as ventricular tachycardia and fibrillation.

Monitoring and Management

When interpreting ECGs of patients on medications, it is crucial to:

- Be aware of the specific drug and its potential effects on the ECG: Understanding the pharmacology and potential ECG changes associated with each medication helps in early detection of drug-induced cardiac effects.

- Monitor electrolyte levels regularly: Especially in patients on diuretics or other drugs that can cause imbalances, regular monitoring of potassium, magnesium, and calcium levels is essential to prevent and manage potential ECG changes.

- Adjust drug dosages as needed: Based on ECG findings and clinical presentation, dosages of medications may need to be adjusted to mitigate adverse effects while ensuring therapeutic efficacy.

- Be vigilant for signs of drug toxicity: Particularly with drugs known to cause significant ECG changes or arrhythmias, close monitoring for symptoms of toxicity (e.g., dizziness, syncope, palpitations) is important.

- Educate patients: Inform patients about the importance of adhering to prescribed medication regimens and attending regular follow-up appointments for monitoring ECG and electrolyte levels.

Understanding the pharmacologic impact on ECG helps in making informed clinical decisions, ensuring patient safety, and optimizing therapeutic outcomes. Accurate interpretation of drug effects on ECG is essential for the effective management of patients on various medications, enabling timely interventions to prevent adverse cardiac events.

DIGITALIS EFFECT

Digitalis, commonly prescribed as digoxin or digitoxin, exerts profound effects on the cardiovascular system, impacting both myocardial contractility and electrical conduction. These effects are crucial to understand when interpreting ECG/EKG readings in patients undergoing digitalis therapy.

Mechanism of Action

Digitalis glycosides inhibit the sodium-potassium ATPase pump (Na+/K+-ATPase) in cardiac myocytes. This inhibition leads to an increase in intracellular sodium concentration, which indirectly affects calcium handling. Specifically, it enhances calcium influx via the sodium-calcium exchanger, resulting in increased intracellular calcium levels. This heightened calcium availability enhances myocardial contractility, making digitalis useful in treating conditions like congestive heart failure.

ECG/EKG Changes Induced by Digitalis

1. PR Interval Prolongation:

Digitalis often prolongs the PR interval on the ECG/EKG. This effect stems from enhanced vagal tone and delayed conduction through the atrioventricular (AV) node. Clinically, this can manifest as first-degree AV block.

2. ST Segment Alterations:

A characteristic ECG finding in patients on digitalis is the "scooping" or "Salvador Dali sign" of the ST segment. This phenomenon involves a downward sloping or sagging appearance of the ST segment, mimicking myocardial ischemia. However, unlike ischemia, it typically does not correlate with coronary artery disease but rather reflects the direct effect of digitalis on myocardial repolarization.

3. T Wave Changes:

Digitalis can cause various alterations in T wave morphology, including flattening, inversion, or even biphasic patterns. These changes are nonspecific but are commonly observed in patients with digitalis toxicity.

4. QT Interval Prolongation:

Prolongation of the QT interval is another potential ECG manifestation of digitalis toxicity. This prolongation can predispose patients to ventricular arrhythmias, particularly torsades de pointes, which is a polymorphic ventricular tachycardia.

5. Arrhythmias:

Despite its use in treating arrhythmias, digitalis can paradoxically induce arrhythmias, especially when levels become toxic. Atrial tachycardias, atrial fibrillation with a slow ventricular response, and ventricular ectopic beats are among the arrhythmias that may occur.

Interpretation Considerations

When interpreting an ECG/EKG of a patient on digitalis therapy, clinicians should consider several factors:

- Baseline ECG: Understanding the patient's baseline ECG characteristics before initiating digitalis treatment helps differentiate new changes from pre-existing ones.

- Digitalis Dosage: Monitoring the dosage and serum levels of digitalis is crucial for detecting potential toxicity early.

- Clinical Context: Integrating ECG findings with clinical symptoms and other diagnostic tests helps differentiate between digitalis effect and other cardiac abnormalities.

Management of Digitalis Effect

Management strategies for digitalis effect on the ECG/EKG include:

- Regular Monitoring: Routine ECG monitoring to detect changes early and assess the response to therapy.

- Dose Adjustment: Adjusting digitalis dosage based on clinical response and ECG findings to maintain therapeutic efficacy while minimizing toxicity.

- Toxicity Management: If digitalis toxicity is suspected, reducing or temporarily discontinuing the medication and providing supportive care are essential steps.

In conclusion, while digitalis glycosides are valuable in managing various cardiac conditions, including heart failure and certain arrhythmias, careful monitoring of their effects on the ECG/EKG is critical. This vigilance ensures that the benefits of digitalis therapy outweigh the potential risks of toxicity, promoting optimal patient care and safety.

ANTIARRHYTHMIC DRUGS

Antiarrhythmic drugs are pharmacological agents used to manage cardiac arrhythmias, which are abnormalities in the rhythm of the heart's electrical activity. These drugs exert their effects by targeting specific ion channels responsible for the generation and propagation of electrical impulses in cardiac cells. Understanding their mechanisms of action is crucial for interpreting their effects on the electrocardiogram (ECG/EKG).

1. Class I Antiarrhythmics act primarily on sodium channels, affecting the phase 0 depolarization of cardiac action potentials. They are further subdivided into three subclasses:

- Class IA drugs (e.g., quinidine, procainamide) prolong the action potential duration by blocking sodium channels and also affect potassium channels. On the ECG, this manifests as prolongation of the QRS complex and the QT interval. Prolonged QT intervals increase the risk of torsades de pointes, a potentially life-threatening arrhythmia.
- Class IB drugs (e.g., lidocaine, mexiletine) shorten the action potential duration by selectively blocking sodium channels, particularly in depolarized cells (those experiencing frequent firing). This results in a narrower QRS complex and a shortened QT interval on the ECG.
- Class IC drugs (e.g., flecainide, propafenone) significantly slow conduction through the atria, ventricles, and His-Purkinje system by blocking sodium channels. This action leads to widened QRS complexes on the ECG but typically does not affect the QT interval significantly.

2. Class II Antiarrhythmics are beta-blockers that primarily block beta-adrenergic receptors in the heart, reducing sympathetic tone and slowing heart rate. They indirectly affect calcium channels, prolonging AV nodal conduction time and resulting in prolonged PR intervals on the ECG. Examples include propranolol and metoprolol.

3. Class III Antiarrhythmics affect potassium channels, delaying repolarization and prolonging the action potential duration.

This class includes drugs like amiodarone and sotalol. Amiodarone, in particular, also has effects on sodium and calcium channels, contributing to its broad-spectrum antiarrhythmic effects. On the ECG, these drugs typically prolong the QT interval, which is a marker of delayed repolarization.

4. Class IV Antiarrhythmics are calcium channel blockers that primarily block L-type calcium channels in cardiac cells, particularly in the AV node. This action slows AV nodal conduction and prolongs the PR interval on the ECG. Verapamil and diltiazem are examples of Class IV antiarrhythmics.

Monitoring the ECG during treatment with antiarrhythmic drugs is essential to assess their efficacy and detect potential adverse effects. Changes in the ECG, such as prolongation of the QT interval or widening of the QRS complex, can indicate the need for dose adjustments or discontinuation of therapy to prevent harmful arrhythmias or other cardiovascular complications. Clinicians must consider each drug's specific indications, contraindications, and potential interactions with other medications to optimize treatment and ensure patient safety.

QT PROLONGATION

QT prolongation on an ECG/EKG refers to an abnormality where the QT interval, which represents the time from the beginning of the QRS complex to the end of the T wave, is lengthened beyond normal limits. The QT interval varies with heart rate, so corrected QT (QTc) is often used for accurate assessment.

Understanding QT Prolongation

The QT interval corresponds to the duration of ventricular depolarization and repolarization. Prolongation can result from various factors:

- Electrolyte Imbalances: Particularly low potassium (hypokalemia) or magnesium levels (hypomagnesemia) can prolong the QT interval.

- Medications: Certain drugs, such as some antibiotics, antiarrhythmics (like amiodarone), antipsychotics (like haloperidol), and antidepressants (like SSRIs), can prolong the QT interval by affecting cardiac repolarization channels (mainly potassium channels).

- Cardiac Conditions: Long QT syndrome (congenital or acquired) is a genetic disorder or can be acquired due to other medical conditions (e.g., myocardial infarction) that predisposes individuals to QT prolongation and potentially life-threatening arrhythmias.

Clinical Significance

Prolonged QT intervals can predispose individuals to serious arrhythmias, most notably Torsades de Pointes, a polymorphic ventricular tachycardia characterized by a twisting pattern on ECG and associated with sudden cardiac death.

ECG/EKG Features

On an ECG/EKG, QT prolongation is identified by measuring the QT interval from the start of the Q wave to the end of the T wave. Typically, a QTc value greater than 450 ms in males and 460 ms in females is considered prolonged. The T wave is usually broadened and may exhibit low-amplitude oscillations or be flattened.

Management

Management of QT prolongation involves:

- Identifying and correcting underlying electrolyte imbalances.

- Adjusting or discontinuing medications known to prolong QT intervals.

- Monitoring ECG changes and electrolyte levels regularly.

- Considering interventions like potassium or magnesium supplementation in severe cases.

QT prolongation on ECG/EKG is a critical finding that requires careful evaluation and management to prevent potentially fatal arrhythmias. Understanding the underlying causes and appropriate management strategies is essential in clinical practice to ensure patient safety and optimal cardiac health.

CHAPTER 7

SPECIAL CONSIDERATIONS

Special Considerations in ECG/EKG interpretation encompass various contexts where the interpretation of electrocardiograms requires specific attention due to unique physiological or pathological conditions. These considerations broaden the scope of ECG analysis beyond typical clinical scenarios, ensuring accurate diagnosis and treatment planning in diverse patient populations.

1. Pediatric ECG/EKG Interpretation: Children present distinct challenges in ECG interpretation due to age-related differences in heart size, rate, and electrical activity. Normal pediatric ECG parameters differ from adults, necessitating familiarity with age-specific norms. Common pediatric arrhythmias, such as sinus arrhythmia and supraventricular tachycardia, require tailored diagnostic approaches.

2. ECG/EKG in Athletes: Athletes often exhibit physiological adaptations, including bradycardia, sinus arrhythmia, and increased vagal tone, which can mimic pathological findings. Differentiating between normal athletic heart changes and abnormal cardiac conditions is crucial for accurate interpretation and appropriate management.

3. ECG/EKG in Pregnancy: Pregnancy induces physiological changes that affect cardiac function and ECG parameters. Normal variations include sinus tachycardia and increased

cardiac output, while conditions like preeclampsia can lead to abnormal ECG findings such as ST segment changes. Monitoring and interpreting ECGs in pregnant women require awareness of these changes to distinguish normal adaptations from potential complications.

Each of these special considerations demands a nuanced approach to ECG interpretation, integrating knowledge of physiological adaptations and pathological conditions specific to each population. This ensures accurate diagnosis and effective management tailored to individual patient needs.

PEDIATRIC ECG/EKG INTERPRETATION

Pediatric ECG interpretation focuses on understanding the electrocardiogram (ECG or EKG) findings in infants, children, and adolescents. Unlike adults, pediatric ECG interpretation requires consideration of age-specific variations in heart rate, rhythm, and morphology of ECG waves.

Basics of Pediatric ECG Interpretation

1. Normal Variations

- Heart Rate: Normal heart rates vary with age, with newborns typically having higher heart rates than older children.
- Rhythm: The sinus node is dominant in pediatric patients, resulting in sinus rhythm being the norm.
- ECG Waves: The size and morphology of ECG waves (P, QRS, T) can differ due to the smaller size of the heart and variations in myocardial conduction pathways.

2. Waveform Characteristics

- P Wave: Typically upright in lead II; abnormal if inverted.
- QRS Complex: Narrower than in adults; duration varies with age.
- T Wave: May be more prominent and asymmetrical compared to adults.

3. Common Pediatric ECG Findings

- Sinus Arrhythmia: Normal in children, where heart rate varies with respiration.
- Junctional Rhythms: More common and often benign in children.
- Prolonged QT Interval: Important to monitor due to risk of arrhythmias.
- T Wave Inversions: Can be normal in young children, but may indicate pathology in older children.

4. Challenges in Interpretation

- Artifact: Movement artifact is more common in infants and young children due to their activity level.
- Lead Placement: Correct lead placement is critical, as small deviations can lead to significant changes in ECG morphology.

5. Clinical Applications

- Screening: ECGs are often used as part of routine screening for congenital heart disease or arrhythmias in newborns and infants.
- Monitoring: Continuous ECG monitoring is crucial in intensive care settings to detect and manage arrhythmias or myocardial ischemia.

Pediatric ECG interpretation requires an understanding of normal age-specific variations in heart rate, rhythm, and ECG morphology. While many principles are similar to adult ECG interpretation, the nuances and specific considerations for pediatric patients ensure accurate diagnosis and appropriate management of cardiac conditions in this population.

AGE-SPECIFIC NORMALS

Age-specific normals in ECG/EKG interpretation refer to the variations in cardiac electrical activity observed across different age groups. These variations are crucial for accurate diagnosis and management, especially in pediatric and geriatric populations.

Pediatric Normals

In infants and children, ECG/EKG findings differ from adults due to anatomical and physiological differences. Key differences include:

- Heart Rate: Higher heart rates are normal in infants and decrease with age.
- QRS Duration: Narrower QRS complexes are typical due to shorter conduction pathways.
- T Wave: May be inverted in lead V1 until adolescence.
- QT Interval: Longer in children, shortens with age.

Adolescents

During adolescence, ECG/EKG findings start resembling adult patterns but may still show:

- Heart Rate: Gradual decrease toward adult rates.
- T Wave: Can still be inverted in some leads without pathology.

Adult Normals

In adults:

- Heart Rate: Generally 60-100 beats per minute at rest.
- QRS Complex: Typically 0.06-0.10 seconds in duration.
- PR Interval: 0.12-0.20 seconds.
- QT Interval: Varies with heart rate, corrected QT (QTc) used for precise assessment.

Geriatric Normals

In older adults:

- Heart Rate: May be lower at rest due to decreased sinoatrial node function.
- P Wave: Increased incidence of atrial enlargement or fibrosis.
- QT Interval: Prolongation due to age-related changes in cardiac conduction.

Clinical Considerations

Understanding age-specific ECG/EKG norms is crucial for distinguishing normal variants from pathological findings. Pediatric ECG/EKG interpretation often requires specialized knowledge to differentiate from congenital abnormalities. In geriatric patients, changes may reflect underlying cardiovascular disease, requiring careful evaluation.

By recognizing age-specific variations in ECG/EKG interpretation, healthcare providers can accurately assess cardiac health across the lifespan and effectively manage cardiovascular conditions.

COMMON PEDIATRIC ARRHYTHMIAS

Pediatric arrhythmias differ from those seen in adults due to the unique anatomical and physiological characteristics of children's hearts. Understanding these differences is crucial for accurate diagnosis and treatment. Common pediatric arrhythmias include both benign and potentially life-threatening conditions.

Types of Pediatric Arrhythmias

Sinus Arrhythmia

Sinus arrhythmia is a normal finding in children and is characterized by a variation in heart rate during the breathing cycle. The heart rate increases during inspiration and decreases during expiration. This type of arrhythmia is generally benign and requires no treatment.

Supraventricular Tachycardia (SVT)

SVT is the most common pathologic arrhythmia in children. It involves an abnormally fast heart rate originating above the ventricles. On an ECG/EKG, SVT typically presents with a rapid heart rate (often >180 bpm in infants and >150 bpm in older children), narrow QRS complexes, and the absence of discernible P waves. SVT can be due to conditions like atrioventricular reentrant tachycardia (AVRT) or atrioventricular nodal reentrant tachycardia (AVNRT).

Atrial Flutter and Atrial Fibrillation

Atrial flutter is less common in children and presents with a sawtooth pattern of atrial waves on the ECG/EKG, often at a rate of 250-350 bpm. Atrial fibrillation, even rarer in pediatrics, shows an irregularly irregular rhythm without distinct P waves.

These conditions usually indicate underlying heart disease or other significant health issues.

Ventricular Tachycardia (VT)

Ventricular tachycardia is rare in children but can be serious. It is characterized by a rapid heart rate originating from the ventricles, with wide QRS complexes on the ECG/EKG. VT in children may be associated with congenital heart defects, myocarditis, or inherited arrhythmia syndromes like long QT syndrome.

Premature Atrial Contractions (PACs) and Premature Ventricular Contractions (PVCs)

PACs and PVCs are common in children and are usually benign. PACs are early beats originating from the atria, seen as early P waves followed by a normal QRS complex. PVCs are early beats originating from the ventricles, characterized by wide, bizarre-looking QRS complexes. Frequent PVCs or those occurring in the presence of underlying heart disease warrant further investigation.

Bradyarrhythmias

Bradyarrhythmias, including sinus bradycardia and atrioventricular (AV) block, are also seen in children. Sinus bradycardia is defined as a slower-than-normal heart rate for the child's age. It can be a normal finding in well-trained athletes but may also result from increased vagal tone or intrinsic sinus node disease. AV block can be congenital or acquired, with varying degrees from first-degree (prolonged PR interval) to third-degree (complete heart block with independent atrial and ventricular rates).

Diagnosis and Management

Diagnosis of pediatric arrhythmias involves a detailed patient history, physical examination, and careful analysis of the ECG/EKG. Further testing, such as Holter monitoring, event recording, and electrophysiological studies, may be necessary for a thorough evaluation.

Management depends on the type and severity of the arrhythmia. Benign arrhythmias like sinus arrhythmia and isolated PACs or PVCs typically require no treatment. SVT and other symptomatic arrhythmias may need pharmacological intervention with medications like beta-blockers or antiarrhythmics, or non-pharmacological treatments such as vagal maneuvers, electrical cardioversion, or catheter ablation.

Understanding the nuances of pediatric arrhythmias on ECG/EKG is essential for appropriate diagnosis and management. With prompt recognition and tailored treatment strategies, most pediatric arrhythmias can be effectively managed, ensuring better outcomes for young patients.

ECG/EKG IN ATHLETES

In athletes, the interpretation of ECG/EKG results requires a nuanced understanding of how regular, intense exercise affects the cardiovascular system. These physiological adaptations, collectively known as "athlete's heart syndrome," encompass a range of changes in heart structure, function, and electrical activity that can manifest on electrocardiograms.

ECG/EKG Characteristics in Athletes

Athletes often exhibit several distinctive ECG/EKG characteristics due to their rigorous training regimen and superior cardiovascular conditioning

1. Bradycardia: Athletes typically demonstrate a lower resting heart rate compared to non-athletes. This bradycardia results from enhanced parasympathetic (vagal) tone and increased myocardial efficiency. A resting heart rate below 60 beats per minute is common and considered normal in well-trained athletes.

2. Increased Vagal Tone: Endurance training enhances vagal tone, leading to a more pronounced resting vagal activity. This can manifest on ECG/EKG as:

- Sinus Bradycardia: A regular, rhythmic heart rate below 60 bpm at rest.
- Increased Sinus Arrhythmia: Athletes often exhibit more significant variation in the RR intervals during normal breathing, reflecting enhanced autonomic modulation.

3. Athlete's Heart Pattern: Long-term athletic training induces specific adaptations in the heart's structure and electrical activity:

- Increased Left Ventricular (LV) Hypertrophy: Due to the demands of endurance training, athletes may develop mild LV hypertrophy. This manifests as increased voltage in the limb leads (especially V5-V6) without evidence of pathological features such as ST-segment depression or T-wave inversion.
- Early Repolarization: Common in athletes, early repolarization is characterized by J-point elevation and concave ST segments in multiple leads, particularly in the inferior and lateral leads. This pattern is typically benign in athletes and does not indicate myocardial ischemia.

4. Ectopic Beats: Athletes may occasionally experience premature atrial or ventricular contractions, which are usually benign and related to heightened vagal tone and enhanced myocardial automaticity.

5. QT Interval: Athletes often exhibit a shorter QT interval due to increased vagal tone and enhanced myocardial repolarization. This adaptation is considered physiological and does not typically predispose to arrhythmias.

Clinical Considerations

When interpreting ECG/EKG results in athletes, healthcare providers must distinguish between normal physiological adaptations and potentially concerning abnormalities that may warrant further evaluation.

- History and Symptoms: Evaluating the athlete's medical history and symptoms is crucial. Symptoms such as syncope, palpitations, or a family history of sudden cardiac death may indicate underlying cardiac pathology rather than benign adaptations.
- Serial ECG/EKGs: Comparing current ECG/EKG results with previous recordings can help identify changes over time, especially concerning new or evolving abnormalities that may require closer monitoring or referral to a specialist.
- Consultation with Cardiologist: In cases where ECG/EKG findings are ambiguous or potentially concerning (e.g., abnormal T wave inversions, significant arrhythmias), consultation with a sports cardiologist or electrophysiologist is recommended. These specialists can provide further evaluation and management tailored to the athlete's specific needs.

Understanding ECG/EKG interpretations in athletes requires recognition of the spectrum of physiological adaptations induced by regular exercise. While many ECG/EKG findings in athletes are benign and reflective of athlete's heart syndrome, healthcare providers must remain vigilant for abnormal findings that may indicate underlying cardiac pathology. Through comprehensive assessment, including history, symptoms, and serial ECG/EKG evaluations, healthcare teams can effectively manage athletes' cardiovascular health and optimize performance while ensuring safety.

PHYSIOLOGICAL CHANGES

Physiological changes in ECG/EKG refer to variations in the electrocardiogram that are considered normal responses to physiological conditions rather than indicators of pathology. These changes can occur due to factors such as age, exercise, body position, and emotional state. Understanding these variations is crucial for accurate interpretation of ECG/EKG readings.

Here are some key physiological changes:

1. Heart Rate: The heart rate can vary widely based on factors like age, fitness level, and emotional state. For example, during exercise or stress, the heart rate typically increases, leading to shorter RR intervals on the ECG/EKG.
2. Rhythm Variability: Normal individuals may exhibit slight irregularities in their heart rhythm, such as sinus arrhythmia, which is a variation in the heart rate that occurs with breathing cycles.
3. P Wave Morphology: The shape and amplitude of the P wave can vary based on the position of the heart within the chest cavity and the angle of lead placement. In healthy individuals, these variations do not indicate pathology.
4. QRS Complex: Changes in the QRS complex can occur with alterations in conduction pathways due to normal anatomical variations or changes in heart position. These changes are typically within normal limits.

5. ST Segment and T Wave: The ST segment can be affected by changes in heart rate and myocardial oxygen demand. T wave morphology can vary with age and electrolyte balance, among other factors, and these variations are usually benign in healthy individuals.
6. QT Interval: The QT interval can vary with heart rate, and slight prolongation or shortening may occur based on autonomic tone and electrolyte balance.
7. Electrolyte Shifts: Physiological changes in electrolyte levels, such as potassium and calcium, can influence the shape and duration of ECG/EKG waves. These changes are typically mild and do not indicate pathological conditions.
8. Body Position: Changes in body position, such as lying down versus standing up, can affect the ECG/EKG due to alterations in venous return and autonomic nervous system activity.
9. Age-Related Changes: Normal aging can lead to subtle changes in ECG/EKG patterns, such as increased P wave duration and PR interval, which reflect age-related changes in conduction pathways and myocardial function.

Understanding these physiological variations is essential for distinguishing normal ECG/EKG changes from pathological findings. Clinicians must consider these factors when interpreting ECG/EKG readings to avoid unnecessary interventions or misdiagnosis based on benign variations in cardiac electrical activity.

DIFFERENTIATING FROM PATHOLOGY

Differentiating normal variants from pathological findings in an ECG/EKG involves a nuanced understanding of cardiac physiology, common clinical conditions, and technical considerations. Here's a detailed exploration:

Normal Variants

1. Sinus Arrhythmia

Sinus arrhythmia is a common finding characterized by variations in heart rate during the respiratory cycle. This physiological variation results from changes in vagal tone during breathing. It typically manifests as a slight increase in heart rate during inspiration and a decrease during expiration. Sinus arrhythmia is benign and often observed in healthy individuals, particularly younger patients.

2. Early Repolarization

Early repolarization refers to an ECG pattern characterized by elevation of the ST segment with a concave upward slope and prominent T waves. This pattern is commonly seen in young, healthy individuals and athletes. It can mimic pathological ST segment elevation, such as that seen in acute myocardial infarction (AMI), but is distinguished by its benign nature and absence of clinical symptoms.

3. Benign Early Repolarization

Benign early repolarization is a variant of early repolarization that typically presents with ST segment elevation in multiple leads, often with notching or slurring at the J point. It is considered a normal variant and does not require specific treatment unless accompanied by clinical symptoms or suggestive history.

Pathological Findings

1. Myocardial Ischemia

Myocardial ischemia results from insufficient blood supply to the heart muscle, often due to coronary artery disease. ECG changes indicative of ischemia include ST segment depression, which may be horizontal or downsloping, and T wave inversion. These changes are typically transient and occur during episodes of ischemia.

2. Myocardial Infarction (MI)

MI occurs when there is prolonged ischemia leading to irreversible damage to the myocardium. The ECG findings depend on the type of MI:

- STEMI (ST-Elevation MI): Characterized by persistent ST segment elevation in contiguous leads, indicating acute transmural myocardial injury.

- Non-STEMI (NSTEMI): May present with ST segment depression, T wave inversion, or no specific ECG changes initially. Diagnosis often relies on cardiac biomarkers and clinical context.

3. Atrial Fibrillation

Atrial fibrillation (AF) is the most common sustained arrhythmia characterized by irregularly irregular ventricular response due to chaotic atrial electrical activity. ECG findings include absent P waves, irregularly spaced QRS complexes, and varying R-R intervals. AF increases the risk of thromboembolic events, particularly stroke, and requires management to control heart rate or rhythm and prevent complications.

4. Ventricular Tachycardia (VT)

VT is a potentially life-threatening arrhythmia characterized by three or more consecutive wide QRS complexes (>120 ms) at a rate >100 bpm. It often presents with hemodynamic compromise and requires prompt intervention, including antiarrhythmic medications, electrical cardioversion, or other advanced cardiac interventions.

5. Heart Block

Heart block refers to impaired conduction between the atria and ventricles. ECG findings include progressive prolongation of the PR interval:

- First-degree AV block: PR interval >200 ms without dropped beats.
- Second-degree AV block: Type I (Wenckebach) and Type II (Mobitz II) patterns involve progressive PR interval prolongation leading to dropped QRS complexes.
- Third-degree AV block (Complete Heart Block): Complete dissociation between atrial and ventricular rhythms, resulting in independent atrial and ventricular rates.

Artifact or Technical Errors

1. Movement Artifact

Movement artifact appears as irregular, sharp fluctuations on the ECG tracing due to patient movement during recording. It can distort waveforms and compromise interpretation.

2. Electrode Misplacement

Incorrect placement of ECG electrodes can lead to altered waveforms or absence of leads, affecting the accuracy of the ECG interpretation. Proper electrode positioning according to standard anatomical landmarks is crucial for obtaining reliable recordings.

3. Lead Reversal

Lead reversal occurs when electrodes are connected incorrectly, resulting in inverted or distorted waveforms. This technical error can lead to misinterpretation of ECG findings and should be corrected promptly to obtain accurate results.

Physiological Adaptations

1. Athlete's Heart

Athletes often exhibit physiological adaptations to regular exercise, including sinus bradycardia, increased vagal tone, and possible benign T wave inversion in inferior and lateral leads. These adaptations reflect the heart's response to increased cardiac output demands and are generally considered normal in athletes without underlying pathology.

2. Pregnancy

Pregnancy induces hormonal and hemodynamic changes that can affect the cardiovascular system. ECG findings in pregnancy may include sinus tachycardia, slight axis deviation, and changes in T wave morphology. These changes are typically physiological responses to pregnancy and do not necessarily indicate pathological conditions.

Drug Effects

1. QT Prolongation

Certain medications, such as antiarrhythmics (e.g., sotalol), antibiotics (e.g., macrolides), and psychotropics (e.g., tricyclic antidepressants), can prolong the QT interval on ECG. Prolonged QT interval increases the risk of torsades de pointes, a potentially life-threatening arrhythmia, and requires careful monitoring and dose adjustments.

2. Digoxin Effect

Digoxin, a medication commonly used in heart failure, can cause characteristic ECG changes known as the digoxin effect. This includes a scooped appearance of the downsloping ST segment and inverted T waves in leads with dominant R waves (e.g., V1-V2). Monitoring serum digoxin levels is essential to prevent toxicity-related arrhythmias.

Pediatric and Geriatric Considerations

1. Pediatric ECG Interpretation

Pediatric ECGs differ from adults due to age-specific heart rate norms, shorter PR intervals, and distinct patterns of congenital heart defects and arrhythmias. Common findings include higher heart rates, normal variants such as pediatric T wave patterns, and specific arrhythmias like supraventricular tachycardia.

2. Geriatric ECG Interpretation

Geriatric patients often exhibit age-related changes in cardiovascular function, including increased prevalence of atrial fibrillation, conduction abnormalities (e.g., bundle branch blocks), and previous myocardial infarctions with associated ECG changes (e.g., Q waves, T wave inversions). These findings necessitate careful assessment and consideration of comorbidities in clinical decision-making.

Accurate interpretation of ECG/EKG findings requires a comprehensive understanding of normal variants, pathological conditions, technical considerations, and physiological adaptations. Clinical correlation with patient history, symptoms, and additional diagnostic tests is essential to differentiate benign findings from those requiring immediate intervention or further investigation. Regular training, familiarity with ECG patterns, and adherence to standardized recording techniques contribute to effective clinical decision-making and patient management.

ECG/EKG IN PREGNANCY

During pregnancy, electrocardiography (ECG or EKG) plays a critical role in assessing and monitoring maternal cardiac health amidst the dynamic physiological changes that occur. These changes are predominantly driven by hormonal shifts, increased blood volume, and adaptations in the cardiovascular system to support the growing fetus.

Physiological Changes

Pregnancy induces significant alterations in cardiovascular function to meet the metabolic demands of both the mother and the developing fetus. Key changes include:

- Increased Blood Volume: Blood volume can increase by up to 50% by mid-pregnancy. This expansion primarily involves plasma volume, which leads to an increase in cardiac output to maintain adequate perfusion.

- Cardiac Structural Changes: The heart undergoes structural adaptations such as dilation of cardiac chambers and thickening of the myocardium. These changes enhance stroke volume and contribute to the increased cardiac output necessary for pregnancy.

- Hormonal Influences: Hormones such as estrogen and progesterone exert profound effects on the cardiovascular system. Estrogen, for example, contributes to vasodilation, while progesterone influences respiratory alkalosis and enhances cardiac output.

Normal ECG Findings

During pregnancy, ECG findings typically reflect these physiological adaptations:

- Heart Rate: Resting heart rate increases by approximately 10-20 beats per minute due to heightened sympathetic activity and hormonal influences. This increase supports the elevated cardiac output needed to meet maternal and fetal metabolic demands.

- Cardiac Axis: The cardiac axis shifts to the left as the uterus enlarges and displaces the diaphragm upwards. This anatomical change alters the orientation of the heart within the chest cavity and affects ECG lead placement and interpretation.

- QT Interval: Prolongation of the QT interval may occur due to hormonal changes, predisposing pregnant women to arrhythmias, particularly in those with underlying susceptibility or electrolyte imbalances.

- T Wave: Inverted T waves in lead III are commonly observed during pregnancy and are generally considered a benign finding. This alteration is attributed to the physiological changes in cardiac conduction pathways.

Common Arrhythmias

While most pregnancies are uncomplicated from a cardiovascular perspective, some women may experience arrhythmias, including:

- Sinus Tachycardia: A physiological response to increased sympathetic tone and metabolic demands. Sinus tachycardia is common during pregnancy and usually benign unless accompanied by symptoms such as palpitations or dizziness.

- Supraventricular Arrhythmias: Conditions like atrial fibrillation or atrial flutter may occur, particularly in women with pre-existing cardiovascular conditions or predisposing factors such as hypertension or structural heart disease.

- Pregnancy-Related Conditions: Gestational hypertension or preeclampsia can lead to electrolyte imbalances and subsequent arrhythmias, necessitating careful monitoring and management.

Clinical Considerations

Managing ECG findings during pregnancy requires a nuanced approach:

- Monitoring: Routine monitoring of maternal ECG may be indicated in high-risk pregnancies or those with pre-existing cardiac conditions. Continuous telemetry or serial ECGs can help detect and manage arrhythmias promptly.

- Treatment: Treatment strategies for arrhythmias in pregnancy focus on symptom management and addressing underlying causes. Non-pharmacological interventions such as lifestyle modifications and electrolyte management are preferred when possible to minimize fetal exposure to medications.

- Collaborative Care: Optimal management involves a multidisciplinary approach, including obstetricians, cardiologists, and specialized healthcare providers. This collaboration ensures comprehensive care tailored to both maternal and fetal needs.

Electrocardiography in pregnancy provides valuable insights into maternal cardiac function amidst the physiological adaptations of gestation. Understanding normal ECG findings and recognizing potential arrhythmias are essential for optimizing maternal health outcomes and ensuring the well-being of the developing fetus. Vigilant monitoring and collaborative management are key to addressing cardiovascular challenges during this transformative period in a woman's life.

NORMAL CHANGES DURING PREGNANCY

During pregnancy, several normal physiological changes can be observed on an electrocardiogram (ECG/EKG) due to the adaptations in the cardiovascular system to support the developing fetus and accommodate the increased maternal metabolic demands. These changes are important to recognize as they can mimic abnormal findings if not understood in the context of pregnancy.

1. Heart Rate: Generally, there is a modest increase in heart rate during pregnancy, primarily due to hormonal influences and increased blood volume. A resting heart rate increase of 10-20 beats per minute can be considered normal.

2. Cardiac Axis: The electrical axis of the heart may shift slightly to the left during pregnancy, which is a normal adaptation to the enlarged uterus displacing the heart.

3. Electrical Changes: There may be mild alterations in the morphology of the ECG/EKG waves, including slight ST segment depression and T wave flattening or inversion, especially in the third trimester. These changes are considered normal unless accompanied by symptoms suggestive of ischemia or other cardiac pathology.

4. QT Interval: The QT interval may be slightly prolonged during pregnancy due to hormonal effects, but significant

prolongation should be monitored closely as it can predispose to arrhythmias.

5. Uterine Contractions: During labor and delivery, uterine contractions can cause transient changes in the ECG/EKG, such as ST segment alterations or T wave changes, which are typically transient and resolve postpartum.

6. Monitoring Considerations: When interpreting ECG/EKG during pregnancy, it's crucial to compare with baseline recordings if available and consider the gestational age of the pregnancy. Consultation with a cardiologist may be necessary if there are significant deviations from these normal changes or if there are concerning symptoms such as chest pain, palpitations, or syncope.

Understanding these normal variations is essential for healthcare providers managing pregnant patients to distinguish between physiological adaptations and pathological conditions affecting the cardiovascular system during pregnancy.

COMMON ARRHYTHMIAS IN PREGNANCY

During pregnancy, the cardiovascular system undergoes significant adaptations to support the growing fetus and increased metabolic demands of the mother. These changes can predispose women to various arrhythmias, ranging from benign sinus tachycardia to more concerning conditions like atrial fibrillation (AF) or higher-degree heart blocks. Understanding these arrhythmias and their implications on electrocardiogram (ECG/EKG) interpretation is crucial for managing maternal health effectively.

Sinus Tachycardia

Sinus tachycardia is a common finding during pregnancy, characterized by a heart rate exceeding 100 bpm at rest. This arrhythmia is primarily due to increased sympathetic tone and hormonal changes, such as elevated levels of catecholamines (e.g., adrenaline) and progesterone. Physiologically, sinus tachycardia helps meet the increased metabolic demands of the mother and fetus. On ECG/EKG, sinus tachycardia appears as regular P waves preceding each QRS complex, with a normal PR interval and QRS duration.

Supraventricular Tachycardias (SVTs)

SVTs, such as paroxysmal supraventricular tachycardia (PSVT), can occur due to abnormal conduction pathways or re-entry circuits within the atria. During pregnancy, SVTs may be more symptomatic due to the physiological changes that increase the risk of arrhythmia initiation. These episodes can lead to palpitations, dizziness, and, in severe cases, compromise maternal cardiac output. On ECG/EKG, SVTs appear as rapid, regular rhythms with narrow QRS complexes and absent or retrograde P waves.

Atrial Fibrillation (AF)

AF is less common during pregnancy but can occur, particularly in women with pre-existing heart conditions such as mitral valve disease or hypertensive disorders. AF is characterized by irregularly irregular ventricular response due to chaotic atrial electrical activity, resulting in an irregularly irregular pulse. On ECG/EKG, AF shows absence of distinct P waves, with irregularly spaced QRS complexes.

Premature Atrial and Ventricular Contractions (PACs/PVCs)

PACs and PVCs are common arrhythmias in healthy individuals but may be more noticeable during pregnancy due to increased awareness of palpitations. PACs arise from ectopic foci in the atria, causing premature beats, often followed by compensatory pauses. PVCs originate from the ventricles and can produce sensations of skipped heartbeats. On ECG/EKG, PACs appear as premature P waves with abnormal morphology relative to sinus beats, while PVCs show wide, bizarre QRS complexes following premature beats.

Heart Block

Heart blocks during pregnancy can range from benign first-degree AV block to more concerning higher-degree blocks. First-degree AV block is characterized by a prolonged PR interval (>200 ms) but typically does not progress to more severe forms. Higher-degree AV blocks (second or third-degree) may occur due to impaired atrioventricular conduction, potentially compromising fetal perfusion. On ECG/EKG, higher-degree AV blocks manifest as progressively prolonged PR intervals with dropped QRS complexes.

Management Considerations

Managing arrhythmias during pregnancy involves a multidisciplinary approach, including obstetricians, cardiologists, and sometimes electrophysiologists. Key considerations include:

- Monitoring: Regular ECG/EKG monitoring may be necessary, especially in high-risk pregnancies or those with known cardiac conditions.

- Symptom Management: Symptomatic arrhythmias may require pharmacological interventions such as beta-blockers or antiarrhythmics. Careful selection of medications is crucial to balance maternal symptom relief with fetal safety.

- Maternal-Fetal Monitoring: Close collaboration between specialties ensures timely intervention if arrhythmias impact maternal hemodynamics or fetal well-being.

- Delivery Planning: Timing and mode of delivery may need adjustment based on maternal cardiac status and arrhythmia stability to minimize risks during labor and postpartum.

Understanding these arrhythmias and their management implications on ECG/EKG interpretation is essential for optimizing maternal and fetal outcomes during pregnancy. Regular assessment and appropriate intervention can mitigate potential complications associated with arrhythmias, ensuring a safe pregnancy and delivery for both mother and baby.

CHAPTER 8
TREATMENT OF ARRHYTHMIAS

Treatment of arrhythmias in ECG/EKG involves various strategies aimed at restoring normal cardiac rhythm and preventing recurrence. These treatments can be broadly categorized into pharmacological and non-pharmacological approaches.

PHARMACOLOGICAL TREATMENT

Pharmacological treatment in ECG/EKG focuses on managing various cardiac arrhythmias using medications that target specific mechanisms of action in the heart's electrical system. These medications are classified as antiarrhythmics and are used to either stabilize cardiac rhythm or control heart rate. Here’s an overview of the pharmacological treatments commonly used:

Antiarrhythmic Medications: These drugs work by altering the electrical properties of cardiac cells to suppress or prevent arrhythmias. They are classified into different classes based on their predominant mechanism of action:

1. Class I (Sodium Channel Blockers): These drugs block sodium channels in cardiac cells, reducing the rate of depolarization and slowing conduction velocity. They are further subdivided into:

- Class IA (e.g., procainamide, disopyramide): Prolong action potential duration and effective refractory period.
- Class IB (e.g., lidocaine, mexiletine): Shorten action potential duration and effective refractory period, used primarily for ventricular arrhythmias.
- Class IC (e.g., flecainide, propafenone): Prolong action potential duration with minimal effect on refractory period.

2. Class II (Beta-Blockers): These drugs block beta-adrenergic receptors, reducing sympathetic nervous system activity and myocardial oxygen demand. They are effective in treating tachyarrhythmias associated with increased sympathetic tone (e.g., atrial fibrillation, atrial flutter).

3. Class III (Potassium Channel Blockers): These drugs prolong the action potential duration and effective refractory period by blocking potassium channels, delaying repolarization. Examples include amiodarone, sotalol, and dofetilide. Amiodarone is particularly versatile, used in both supraventricular and ventricular arrhythmias, but has significant side effects.

4. Class IV (Calcium Channel Blockers): These drugs block calcium channels in cardiac cells, reducing calcium influx during depolarization. They are effective in slowing atrioventricular conduction and controlling heart rate in conditions such as atrial fibrillation and atrial flutter. Examples include verapamil and diltiazem.

Rate Control vs. Rhythm Control

- Rate Control: Focuses on slowing the heart rate to a more normal range (typically less than 100 beats per minute at rest) without necessarily converting the arrhythmia to sinus rhythm. Beta-blockers and calcium channel blockers are commonly used for rate control.

- Rhythm Control: Aimed at restoring sinus rhythm and maintaining it. It involves cardioversion (either electrical or pharmacological) to terminate the arrhythmia and maintain sinus rhythm thereafter. Antiarrhythmic drugs from various classes are used for rhythm control, often based on the type and severity of the arrhythmia.

Considerations

- Side Effects and Monitoring: Antiarrhythmic medications can have significant side effects, including proarrhythmia (paradoxical worsening of arrhythmias), electrolyte disturbances, and organ toxicity (especially with drugs like amiodarone). Close monitoring of electrocardiograms (ECGs), electrolytes, and renal/liver function is crucial during treatment.

- Individualized Therapy: Selection of antiarrhythmic therapy is highly individualized, considering factors such as the type of arrhythmia, patient comorbidities, drug interactions, and potential adverse effects.

Pharmacological treatment in ECG/EKG interpretation involves a nuanced understanding of these medications' mechanisms, indications, and potential risks to effectively manage and improve patient outcomes in cardiac arrhythmias.

ANTIARRHYTHMIC MEDICATIONS

Antiarrhythmic medications are used to manage and treat arrhythmias by influencing the electrical activity of the heart. These medications can affect various aspects of the cardiac action potential and conduction system, which are often reflected in ECG/EKG changes. Understanding these changes is crucial for clinicians to monitor therapeutic effects and potential side effects.

Classes of Antiarrhythmic Medications

Antiarrhythmic medications are classified into four main classes based on the Vaughan-Williams classification system:

Class I: Sodium Channel Blockers

Class I drugs block sodium channels, reducing the rate of depolarization in phase 0 of the action potential. This class is subdivided into three groups based on their effect on the action potential duration:

- Class IA (e.g., Quinidine, Procainamide, Disopyramide): These drugs moderate sodium channel blockade and prolong the action potential. They can widen the QRS complex and prolong the QT interval.

- Class IB (e.g., Lidocaine, Mexiletine): These drugs have a weak sodium channel blockade and shorten the action potential duration. They primarily affect ischemic or depolarized tissues with minimal ECG changes.

- Class IC (e.g., Flecainide, Propafenone): These drugs have a strong sodium channel blockade with little effect on the action potential duration. They significantly widen the QRS complex.

Class II: Beta Blockers

Beta blockers (e.g., Metoprolol, Atenolol, Propranolol) inhibit the effects of sympathetic stimulation by blocking beta-adrenergic receptors. They reduce heart rate, decrease AV node conduction, and lower myocardial contractility. ECG changes include a decrease in heart rate and a prolonged PR interval.

Class III: Potassium Channel Blockers

Class III drugs (e.g., Amiodarone, Sotalol, Dofetilide) block potassium channels, prolonging repolarization and the duration of the action potential. This results in a prolonged QT interval. Amiodarone, the most commonly used drug in this class, can also cause bradycardia and AV block due to its effects on sodium and calcium channels.

Class IV: Calcium Channel Blockers

Calcium channel blockers (e.g., Verapamil, Diltiazem) inhibit the influx of calcium ions during phase 2 of the action potential. They are effective in slowing AV node conduction and reducing heart rate, which is reflected in a prolonged PR interval on the ECG. These drugs are particularly useful in treating supraventricular tachycardias.

Other Antiarrhythmic Medications

Adenosine

Adenosine is a nucleoside that activates adenosine receptors, leading to hyperpolarization of the AV node and transient heart block. It is used for the acute termination of paroxysmal supraventricular tachycardia (PSVT). On the ECG, adenosine causes a transient asystole followed by the restoration of normal sinus rhythm.

Digoxin

Digoxin enhances vagal tone and inhibits the sodium-potassium ATPase pump, leading to increased intracellular calcium. It slows AV node conduction, making it useful in controlling ventricular rate in atrial fibrillation. ECG changes include a prolonged PR interval, decreased heart rate, and characteristic "scooping" of the ST segment known as the "digoxin effect."

Magnesium Sulfate

Magnesium sulfate is used in the treatment of torsades de pointes and other arrhythmias associated with hypomagnesemia. It helps stabilize the cardiac membrane and can correct prolonged QT intervals caused by electrolyte imbalances.

Monitoring and Safety

Close monitoring of the ECG is essential when initiating or adjusting antiarrhythmic therapy to detect therapeutic effects and potential adverse reactions. Key aspects to monitor include:

- Heart Rate and Rhythm: To ensure the medication is effectively controlling the arrhythmia without causing bradycardia or new arrhythmias.

- PR Interval: Prolongation may indicate AV nodal block, especially with beta blockers, calcium channel blockers, and digoxin.

- QRS Complex Duration: Widening of the QRS complex, particularly with Class I drugs, can signal excessive sodium channel blockade.

- QT Interval: Prolongation is a significant concern with Class IA and III drugs as it can predispose to torsades de pointes, a potentially life-threatening arrhythmia.

Adjustments in dosing, discontinuation of the medication, or switching to an alternative therapy may be necessary based on ECG findings and clinical assessment. Regular follow-up and patient education on the signs and symptoms of arrhythmias and adverse effects are crucial for safe and effective management.

RATE CONTROL VS. RHYTHM CONTROL

In the management of arrhythmias, particularly atrial fibrillation (AF), two primary strategies are employed: rate control and rhythm control. Both approaches aim to alleviate symptoms and prevent complications, but they differ fundamentally in their objectives and methods.

Rate Control

Rate control focuses on controlling the heart rate without necessarily restoring the normal sinus rhythm. This approach is often preferred for patients who are asymptomatic or have mild symptoms, especially if they have persistent or permanent AF. The goal is to maintain the ventricular rate within an acceptable range to prevent tachycardia-induced cardiomyopathy and to improve symptoms.

Medications for Rate Control

1. Beta-Blockers: These drugs, such as metoprolol and atenolol, reduce the heart rate by blocking the effects of adrenaline on the heart.

2. Calcium Channel Blockers: Non-dihydropyridine calcium channel blockers like diltiazem and verapamil slow the heart rate by inhibiting calcium influx into cardiac cells.

3. Digoxin: This medication enhances vagal tone and slows conduction through the atrioventricular (AV) node, reducing the heart rate, particularly at rest.

Advantages of Rate Control

i. Simplicity and lower risk: Rate control is often easier to achieve and maintain, with fewer risks compared to rhythm control.
ii. Suitable for older patients: Rate control is generally recommended for older patients or those with comorbidities that make rhythm control less feasible.

Disadvantages of Rate Control

i. Persistent arrhythmia: The underlying atrial fibrillation remains, which can be associated with ongoing symptoms in some patients.
ii. Anticoagulation: Patients still require anticoagulation to prevent thromboembolism due to the continued presence of AF.

Rhythm Control

Rhythm control aims to restore and maintain the normal sinus rhythm. This strategy is often pursued in patients with symptomatic AF, those with a first episode of AF, or younger patients without significant structural heart disease.

Methods for Rhythm Control

1. Antiarrhythmic Medications: Drugs like amiodarone, flecainide, and sotalol are used to restore and maintain sinus rhythm.

2. Electrical Cardioversion: This procedure involves delivering a synchronized electrical shock to the heart to reset the rhythm back to normal.

3. Ablation Therapy: Catheter ablation targets specific areas in the heart to disrupt the abnormal electrical pathways causing AF. Pulmonary vein isolation is a common ablation procedure for AF.

4. Surgical Options: In some cases, surgical procedures like the maze procedure are employed to create scar tissue that interrupts the electrical signals causing AF.

Advantages of Rhythm Control

i. Symptom relief: Many patients experience significant improvement in symptoms and quality of life when sinus rhythm is restored.

ii. Potential for normal heart function: Restoring sinus rhythm can improve hemodynamic function and prevent AF-related complications such as heart failure.

Disadvantages of Rhythm Control

i. Recurrence: AF often recurs despite attempts to maintain sinus rhythm, necessitating repeated interventions.

ii. Side effects and risks: Antiarrhythmic medications and procedures like ablation carry risks of adverse effects and complications.

Choosing Between Rate and Rhythm Control

The decision between rate control and rhythm control is individualized, taking into account the patient's symptoms, the duration and type of AF, underlying heart disease, comorbid conditions, and patient preferences. In some cases, a combination of both strategies may be used, starting with rhythm control and transitioning to rate control if rhythm control fails.

Clinical guidelines often recommend rate control as the initial strategy for many patients, particularly those who are older or have minimal symptoms. Rhythm control is typically considered for younger patients, those with significant symptoms, or those for whom rate control is ineffective.

Both rate control and rhythm control have their roles in the management of atrial fibrillation and other arrhythmias. The choice between them depends on various factors, including patient characteristics, symptom burden, and risk profiles. Effective management often involves a patient-centered approach, considering both the clinical and lifestyle impacts of each strategy.

NON-PHARMACOLOGICAL TREATMENT

Non-pharmacological treatment in ECG/EKG refers to interventions used to manage and treat arrhythmias that do not involve medications. These treatments include electrical cardioversion, ablation therapy, and implantable devices such as pacemakers and implantable cardioverter-defibrillators (ICDs).

1. Electrical Cardioversion: A procedure that uses a controlled electrical shock to restore a normal heart rhythm in patients with certain arrhythmias.

2. Ablation Therapy: A technique that uses energy (radiofrequency or cryothermal) to destroy specific areas of heart tissue causing abnormal electrical signals, thereby restoring normal rhythm.

3. Implantable Devices:

- Pacemakers: Devices implanted under the skin to stimulate the heart to beat at a normal rate and rhythm, typically used for slow heart rates or heart block.

- Implantable Cardioverter-Defibrillators (ICDs): Devices that deliver a high-energy shock to correct life-threatening arrhythmias such as ventricular tachycardia or ventricular fibrillation.

- Cardiac Resynchronization Therapy (CRT): Specialized pacemakers used to improve heart function in patients with heart failure by coordinating the contractions of the heart's ventricles.

ELECTRICAL CARDIOVERSION

Electrical cardioversion is a medical procedure used to restore a normal heart rhythm in patients experiencing certain types of abnormal heartbeats, such as atrial fibrillation, atrial flutter, or supraventricular tachycardia. This procedure involves delivering a controlled electric shock to the heart through the chest wall, which helps to reset the heart's electrical activity and return it to a normal rhythm.

Indications for Electrical Cardioversion

Electrical cardioversion is typically indicated for patients who have arrhythmias that are symptomatic, hemodynamically unstable, or refractory to medication.

Common conditions that may require electrical cardioversion include:

i. Atrial Fibrillation (AFib): This is a common type of irregular heartbeat that can lead to blood clots, stroke, heart failure, and other heart-related complications. Cardioversion can help restore a normal rhythm and improve symptoms.
ii. Atrial Flutter: Similar to atrial fibrillation but usually more regular, atrial flutter can also cause similar symptoms and risks.
iii. Supraventricular Tachycardia (SVT): A rapid heart rate originating above the ventricles can sometimes be corrected with electrical cardioversion.
iv. Ventricular Tachycardia (VT) with a Pulse: In certain cases, this life-threatening arrhythmia can be treated with cardioversion.

Preparation for Electrical Cardioversion

Before the procedure, several steps are taken to ensure patient safety and effectiveness:

i. Assessment: A thorough medical history, physical examination, and diagnostic tests, including an ECG/EKG, are performed to identify the type and cause of the arrhythmia.
ii. Anticoagulation Therapy: Patients with atrial fibrillation or flutter may need to take anticoagulants for several weeks before the procedure to reduce the risk of blood clots and stroke.
iii. Fasting: Patients are usually instructed to fast for at least 6-8 hours before the procedure to reduce the risk of aspiration during sedation.
iv. Intravenous (IV) Access: An IV line is placed for administering medications and fluids.

The Procedure

Electrical cardioversion is typically performed in a hospital setting under sedation to minimize discomfort. The steps of the procedure include:

i. Sedation: The patient is given sedative or anesthetic medications through the IV to ensure they are comfortable and pain-free during the procedure.
ii. Placement of Electrodes: Patches or paddles connected to a defibrillator are placed on the patient's chest, and sometimes on the back, to deliver the shock.
iii. Synchronization: The defibrillator is set to deliver the shock in sync with the heart's electrical activity to avoid

inducing ventricular fibrillation, a potentially life-threatening condition.

iv. Delivery of Shock: One or more shocks are delivered to the heart to reset its electrical activity. The defibrillator monitors the heart rhythm and guides the delivery of the shock at the optimal moment.

Post-Procedure Care

After cardioversion, the patient is monitored to ensure the heart has returned to a normal rhythm and to check for any complications:

i. Monitoring: The patient's heart rhythm, blood pressure, and oxygen levels are continuously monitored for a period after the procedure.
ii. Assessment: The effectiveness of the cardioversion is assessed using ECG/EKG and clinical evaluation.
iii. Follow-Up: The patient may need follow-up visits to adjust medications, manage any underlying conditions, and monitor for recurrence of arrhythmia.

Potential Complications

Although generally safe, electrical cardioversion carries some risks, including:

i. Skin Burns: Mild burns can occur at the sites where the electrodes were placed.
ii. Arrhythmias: In rare cases, the procedure can cause new or more severe arrhythmias.
iii. Stroke: If blood clots are present in the heart, they can be dislodged during cardioversion, leading to a stroke. This is why anticoagulation therapy is crucial beforehand.

iv. Hemodynamic Instability: Temporary drops in blood pressure or other cardiac complications can occur.

Electrical cardioversion is a highly effective procedure for restoring normal heart rhythm in patients with certain types of arrhythmias. With proper preparation, execution, and post-procedure care, the risks can be minimized, making it a valuable tool in the management of arrhythmias. The involvement of a skilled medical team and appropriate use of anticoagulation therapy are key components in ensuring a successful outcome.

ABLATION THERAPY

Ablation therapy is a medical procedure used to treat certain types of cardiac arrhythmias, which are irregular heartbeats that can be detected and diagnosed using an ECG/EKG. This therapy involves the use of heat (radiofrequency energy) or extreme cold (cryotherapy) to create small scars in the heart tissue. These scars disrupt abnormal electrical pathways, thereby restoring normal rhythm.

Indications for Ablation Therapy

Ablation therapy is typically recommended for patients who have not responded to medications or for those who experience significant side effects from antiarrhythmic drugs. It is commonly used to treat a variety of arrhythmias, including atrial fibrillation, atrial flutter, supraventricular tachycardia (SVT), and some forms of ventricular tachycardia.

Types of Ablation

There are several types of ablation, depending on the technology used:

- Radiofrequency Ablation (RFA): This is the most common form, using high-frequency electrical currents to generate heat and create scar tissue.

- Cryoablation: This technique uses extreme cold to freeze and destroy abnormal heart tissue.

- Laser Ablation: This method uses laser energy to ablate tissue, though it is less commonly used than RFA and cryoablation.

Procedure

Ablation therapy is usually performed in a cardiac electrophysiology lab by a specialized cardiologist known as an electrophysiologist. The procedure involves the following steps:

- Preparation: The patient is sedated or given general anesthesia. Electrodes are placed on the chest to monitor the heart's activity.

- Catheter Insertion: A catheter, a thin flexible tube, is inserted through a vein in the groin, neck, or arm and guided to the heart using fluoroscopy, a type of X-ray imaging.

- Mapping: The electrophysiologist uses specialized equipment to map the heart's electrical activity and identify the area(s) causing the arrhythmia.

- Ablation: Once the abnormal area is identified, the catheter delivers either radiofrequency energy or cryotherapy to ablate the tissue.

- Verification: After ablation, the electrophysiologist re-maps the heart to ensure the abnormal pathway has been successfully disrupted.

- Recovery: The catheter is removed, and the insertion site is closed. The patient is monitored for a few hours to ensure there are no immediate complications.

Effectiveness and Risks

Ablation therapy is highly effective for many types of arrhythmias, with success rates varying depending on the specific condition treated. For example, it has a high success rate in treating atrial flutter and certain types of SVT. However, the success rate for atrial fibrillation may be lower, and some patients might require multiple procedures.

Like any medical procedure, ablation carries risks, although they are generally low. Potential complications include bleeding, infection, damage to blood vessels, heart valve damage, and in rare cases, stroke or heart attack. Long-term, patients might experience arrhythmia recurrence, necessitating further treatment.

Post-Procedure Care

After the procedure, patients are typically advised to rest and avoid strenuous activities for a few days. Follow-up appointments are crucial to monitor the heart's rhythm and ensure the ablation was successful. Medications may still be required initially, but many patients can reduce or discontinue their use over time.

Ablation therapy is a valuable treatment option for patients with certain cardiac arrhythmias. By disrupting abnormal electrical pathways in the heart, it can restore normal rhythm and improve quality of life. While it carries some risks, its high success rate and potential to reduce the need for long-term medication make it a widely used and effective treatment. Regular follow-up and monitoring are essential to ensure lasting benefits and address any complications that may arise.

IMPLANTABLE DEVICES (PACEMAKERS, ICDS)

Pacemakers

A pacemaker is a small device implanted in the chest or abdomen to help control abnormal heart rhythms. This device uses electrical pulses to prompt the heart to beat at a normal rate. Pacemakers are often used to treat bradycardia (slow heart rate) or heart block (a problem with the heart's electrical conduction system).

Components of a Pacemaker

i. Pulse Generator: This is the small metal case that contains the battery and the electrical circuitry that regulates the rate of electrical pulses sent to the heart.
ii. Leads (Electrodes): These are insulated wires that carry the electrical pulses from the pulse generator to the heart muscle.

Types of Pacemakers:

i. Single-Chamber Pacemaker: This type has one lead placed in either the right atrium or the right ventricle of the heart.
ii. Dual-Chamber Pacemaker: This type has two leads, one placed in the right atrium and one in the right ventricle. It helps coordinate the timing between the atrium and the ventricle.

iii. Biventricular Pacemaker: This type, also known as cardiac resynchronization therapy (CRT), has three leads placed in the right atrium, right ventricle, and left ventricle. It is used in patients with heart failure to help improve the heart's efficiency.

ECG/EKG Appearance

- Pacing Spikes: The most distinctive feature of a pacemaker on an ECG/EKG is the presence of pacing spikes. These are small, sharp vertical lines that precede the paced cardiac depolarization.

- Capture: Following a pacing spike, a corresponding P wave (atrial pacing) or QRS complex (ventricular pacing) should be observed, indicating that the heart muscle has responded to the electrical stimulus.

- Fusion and Pseudofusion Beats: These occur when the heart's natural pacemaker and the implanted pacemaker both contribute to the heart's activity, resulting in a combined waveform.

Implantable Cardioverter-Defibrillators (ICDs)

An ICD is a device designed to monitor heart rhythms and deliver electrical shocks when it detects dangerous arrhythmias, such as ventricular tachycardia or ventricular fibrillation. ICDs are critical for preventing sudden cardiac death in patients with a high risk of life-threatening arrhythmias.

Components of an ICD

i. Pulse Generator: Similar to a pacemaker, the pulse generator contains the battery and circuitry, but it also includes a capacitor capable of delivering a high-energy shock.

ii. Leads: These wires are positioned within the heart and can deliver both low-energy pacing impulses and high-energy shocks.

Functions of an ICD

i. Antitachycardia Pacing (ATP): The ICD can deliver a series of rapid pacing pulses to interrupt a tachycardia.
ii. Cardioversion: The ICD can deliver a synchronized shock to terminate an abnormal rhythm and restore normal heart rhythm.
iii. Defibrillation: For very rapid and chaotic rhythms like ventricular fibrillation, the ICD delivers a high-energy shock to reset the heart's electrical activity.

ECG/EKG Appearance

- Pacing and Sensing: Similar to a pacemaker, ICDs can pace the heart and show pacing spikes on the ECG/EKG.

- Shock Delivery: If the ICD delivers a shock, this is often seen as a large, abrupt deflection on the ECG/EKG, followed by a return to a normal or near-normal rhythm.

- Post-Shock Monitoring: After a shock, the ICD monitors the heart rhythm to ensure the arrhythmia is terminated and may adjust its pacing if necessary.

Clinical Considerations

- Lead Placement and Malfunction: Proper lead placement is crucial for the device's effectiveness. Malfunction or lead displacement can lead to inappropriate pacing or failure to deliver necessary shocks.

- Battery Life and Device Longevity: Both pacemakers and ICDs require periodic checks to monitor battery life and device functionality. The average lifespan of these devices ranges from 5 to 15 years, depending on usage.

- Patient Monitoring: Patients with pacemakers and ICDs require regular follow-up to ensure the device is functioning correctly and to make any necessary adjustments.

Pacemakers and ICDs are vital tools in managing patients with arrhythmias and preventing sudden cardiac death. Understanding their function and interpretation on an ECG/EKG is essential for healthcare providers to ensure optimal patient care and timely intervention when needed.

EMERGENCY MANAGEMENT OF ARRHYTHMIAS

Emergency management of arrhythmias in ECG/EKG involves swift and decisive actions aimed at stabilizing the patient and restoring normal cardiac rhythm to prevent potential cardiac arrest or further complications. The approach varies depending on the type of arrhythmia observed.

For ventricular tachycardia (VT) and ventricular fibrillation (VF), immediate intervention is critical. These arrhythmias can rapidly degenerate into cardiac arrest. Defibrillation is the primary intervention for VF and pulseless VT. It involves delivering a shock to the heart to interrupt the chaotic electrical activity, allowing the heart to reestablish an organized rhythm.

In cases of supraventricular tachycardias (SVT) like atrial fibrillation (AF) or atrial flutter, the management focuses on rate control and symptom management. This often includes administering medications such as beta-blockers, calcium channel blockers, or digoxin to slow down the heart rate and improve hemodynamics.

For bradycardias associated with hemodynamic instability or symptomatic patients, transcutaneous pacing may be initiated. This involves placing external pacing pads on the patient's chest and delivering electrical impulses to stimulate the heart to beat at a desired rate.

In cases where pharmacological interventions are warranted, medications such as adenosine may be administered for certain types of SVT to transiently block conduction through the AV node, thereby terminating the arrhythmia. Amiodarone or lidocaine may be used for stabilizing ventricular arrhythmias in non-arrest situations.

Advanced cardiac life support (ACLS) protocols guide these interventions, emphasizing the importance of effective chest compressions, airway management, and appropriate drug administration based on the specific rhythm identified on the ECG/EKG.

Throughout the management of arrhythmias, continuous monitoring of the patient's cardiac rhythm and vital signs is crucial. This allows for timely recognition of changes or recurrence of arrhythmias, facilitating prompt adjustment of treatment strategies as needed.

ADVANCED CARDIAC LIFE SUPPORT (ACLS) PROTOCOLS

Advanced Cardiac Life Support (ACLS) protocols are critical guidelines used in the management of cardiac arrest and other cardiovascular emergencies. These protocols involve a series of systematic interventions aimed at restoring and maintaining effective circulation and cardiac function in patients experiencing life-threatening arrhythmias or cardiac arrest.

ACLS protocols in ECG/EKG interpretation primarily focus on identifying and managing specific cardiac rhythms and associated conditions.

Key components include:

- Recognition of Arrhythmias: ACLS emphasizes the rapid identification and interpretation of cardiac rhythms through ECG/EKG monitoring. This involves distinguishing between shockable rhythms (e.g., ventricular fibrillation, pulseless ventricular tachycardia) and non-shockable rhythms (e.g., asystole, pulseless electrical activity).

- Immediate Interventions: Based on the identified rhythm, ACLS provides immediate interventions such as defibrillation for shockable rhythms or initiation of CPR for non-shockable rhythms. Defibrillation aims to restore a perfusing rhythm by delivering an electric shock to the heart during ventricular fibrillation or pulseless ventricular tachycardia.

- Medication Administration: ACLS protocols outline the administration of specific medications to stabilize cardiac rhythms and improve circulation. Medications may include antiarrhythmic agents (e.g., amiodarone, lidocaine), vasopressors (e.g., epinephrine), and adjunctive therapies (e.g., magnesium sulfate for torsades de pointes).

- Post-Resuscitation Care: ACLS extends beyond the immediate resuscitation phase to include post-resuscitation care strategies. This involves optimizing ventilation and oxygenation, monitoring for recurrent arrhythmias or complications, and ensuring appropriate hemodynamic support.

- Team Coordination and Communication: Effective ACLS implementation requires coordinated efforts among healthcare providers, emphasizing clear roles, effective communication, and adherence to standardized protocols. Team dynamics and leadership play a crucial role in optimizing outcomes during resuscitation efforts.

- Integration with ECG/EKG Findings: Throughout ACLS interventions, continuous ECG/EKG monitoring guides decision-making regarding the effectiveness of interventions, the need for rhythm reassessment, and adjustments in therapy as indicated by evolving cardiac rhythms.

ACLS protocols in ECG/EKG interpretation are designed to facilitate timely and systematic management of cardiac emergencies. By integrating advanced cardiovascular life support principles with real-time ECG/EKG interpretation, healthcare providers can improve the chances of successful resuscitation and patient outcomes in critical situations.

DEFIBRILLATION AND CPR

Defibrillation and CPR are critical interventions in managing cardiac emergencies, particularly in the context of ECG/EKG interpretation and arrhythmia management.

Defibrillation

Defibrillation is a procedure used to restore normal heart rhythm in cases of life-threatening arrhythmias, particularly ventricular fibrillation (VF) and pulseless ventricular tachycardia (VT). These arrhythmias can cause the heart to quiver ineffectively, leading to a cessation of effective circulation (cardiac arrest).

During defibrillation, an electrical shock is delivered to the heart using a defibrillator. The shock briefly stops all electrical activity in the heart, allowing the natural pacemaker cells of the heart to reestablish a normal rhythm. This procedure is typically performed using pads or paddles placed on the chest, and it is crucial that it is administered promptly to maximize the chance of restoring normal heart function.

Cardiopulmonary Resuscitation (CPR)

CPR is a lifesaving technique used when someone's heartbeat or breathing has stopped. It involves a combination of chest compressions and rescue breaths to manually circulate oxygenated blood to vital organs, especially the brain and heart, until further medical help arrives.

In the context of ECG/EKG, CPR is initiated immediately upon identifying cardiac arrest or non-responsiveness of the patient. High-quality CPR involves:

- Chest Compressions: These are performed to manually pump blood through the heart to maintain circulation. Proper technique involves pressing down firmly and rapidly on the center of the chest, between the nipples, to a depth of at least 2 inches (5 cm) in adults.

- Rescue Breaths: Oxygen is delivered to the patient's lungs through rescue breaths, which help maintain oxygenation of the blood.

The integration of defibrillation with CPR is critical in managing cardiac arrest. For ventricular fibrillation or pulseless ventricular tachycardia detected on the ECG/EKG, immediate CPR followed by prompt defibrillation significantly increases the chances of survival. CPR helps to maintain minimal blood flow to vital organs until defibrillation can be performed, potentially restoring a normal heart rhythm and improving overall outcomes.

Overall, understanding and promptly implementing defibrillation and CPR based on ECG/EKG findings are essential skills for healthcare providers in managing cardiac emergencies and improving patient survival rates.

REFERENCES

Dubin, D. (2000). *Rapid Interpretation of EKG's: An Interactive Course.* Cover Publishing Company.

Marriott, H. J. L. (2007). *Marriott's Practical Electrocardiography.* Lippincott Williams & Wilkins.

Garcia, T. B., & Miller, G. T. (2013). *Arrhythmia Recognition: The Art of Interpretation.* Jones & Bartlett Learning.

Goldberger, A. L. (2012). *Clinical Electrocardiography: A Simplified Approach.* Elsevier Saunders.

Wagner, G. S. (2008). *Marriott's Practical Electrocardiography.* Lippincott Williams & Wilkins.

Bayés de Luna, A. (2012). *Clinical Electrocardiography: A Textbook.* Wiley-Blackwell.

Antman, E. M., et al. (2004). ACC/AHA Guidelines for the Management of Patients With ST-Elevation Myocardial Infarction. *Journal of the American College of Cardiology,* 44(3), E1-E211.

Surawicz, B., & Knilans, T. K. (2008). *Chou's Electrocardiography in Clinical Practice: Adult and Pediatric.* Saunders.

Josephson, M. E. (2008). *Clinical Cardiac Electrophysiology: Techniques and Interpretations.* Lippincott Williams & Wilkins.

Rautaharju, P. M., et al. (2009). AHA/ACCF/HRS Recommendations for the Standardization and Interpretation of the Electrocardiogram: Part IV: The ST Segment, T and U Waves, and the QT Interval. *Circulation,* 119(10), e241-e250.

Kass, R. S., & Clancy, C. E. (2006). The Mechanisms of Sudden Cardiac Death Related to Drugs. *Journal of Clinical Investigation,* 116(8), 1974-1984.

Zipes, D. P., & Jalife, J. (2013). *Cardiac Electrophysiology: From Cell to Bedside.* Saunders.

Braunwald, E. (2008). *Braunwald's Heart Disease: A Textbook of Cardiovascular Medicine.* Saunders.

Wellen, H. J. V. (2013). *The ECG in Emergency Decision Making.* Elsevier.

Camm, A. J., et al. (2010). Guidelines for the Management of Atrial Fibrillation. *European Heart Journal,* 31(19), 2369-2429.

Alpert, J. S., & Thygesen, K. (2007). Myocardial Infarction Redefined—A Consensus Document of The Joint European Society of Cardiology/American College of Cardiology Committee for the Redefinition of Myocardial Infarction. *Journal of the American College of Cardiology,* 36(3), 959-969.

American Heart Association (2020). *2020 American Heart Association Guidelines for CPR and ECC.* American Heart Association.

Davies, M. J., et al. (2010). The Pathology of the Coronary Atherosclerotic Plaque. *Heart,* 83(3), 361-366.

Smith, S. W. (2014). *The ECG in Acute MI: An Evidence-Based Manual of Reperfusion Therapy.* Wiley-Blackwell.

Chhabra, L., & Devadoss, R. (2014). Significance of Electrocardiographic Leads. *Journal of the American College of Cardiology*, 63(4), 400-403.

APPENDIX

Cheat Sheet for ECG/EKG Interpretation

Arrhythmias	Description	Causes	Treatment
Sinus Arrhythmia 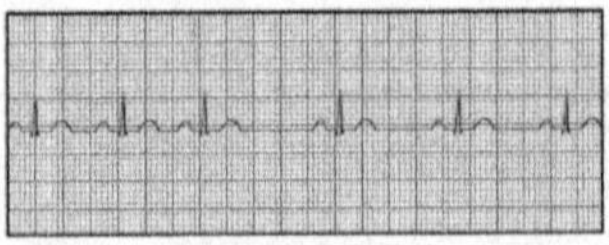	• Irregular atrial and ventricular rhythms. • Normal P wave preceding each QRS complex.	• Normal variation of normal sinus rhythm in athletes, children, and the elderly. • Can be seen in digoxin toxicity and inferior wall MI.	• Atropine if rate decreases below 40bpm.
Sinus Tachycardia 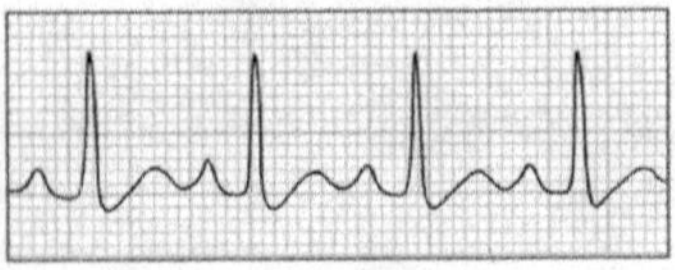	• Atrial and ventricular rhythms are regular. • Rate > 100 bpm. • Normal P wave preceding each QRS complex.	• Normal physiologic response to fever, exercise, anxiety, dehydration, or pain. • May accompany shock, left-sided heart failure, cardiac tamponade, hyperthyroidism, and anemia. • Atropine, epinephrine, quinidine, caffeine, nicotine, and alcohol use.	• Correction of underlying cause. • Beta-adrenergic blockers or calcium channel blockers for symptomatic patients.
Sinus Bradycardia 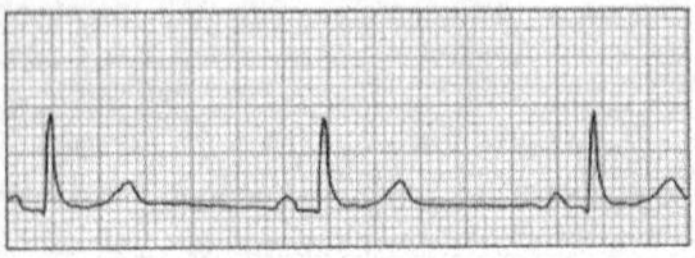	• Regular atrial and ventricular rhythms. • Rate < 60 bpm. • Normal P wave preceding each QRS complex.	• Normal in a well-conditioned heart (e.g., athletes). • Increased intracranial pressure; increased vagal tone due to straining during defecation, vomiting, intubation, mechanical ventilation.	• Follow ACLS protocol for administration of atropine for symptoms of low cardiac output, dizziness, weakness, altered LOC, or low blood pressure. • Pacemaker
Sinoatrial (SA) arrest or block 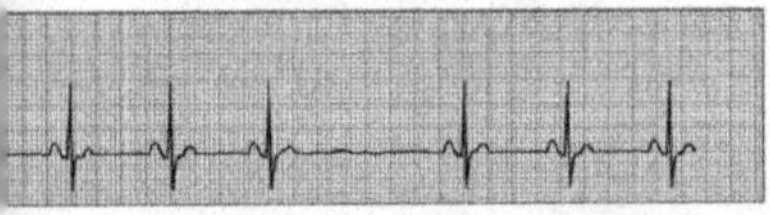	• Atrial and ventricular rhythms are normal except for missing complexes. • Normal P wave preceding each QRS complex. • Pause not equal to multiple of the previous rhythm.	• Infection • Coronary artery disease, degenerative heart disease, acute inferior wall MI. • Vagal stimulation, Valsalva's maneuver, carotid sinus massage.	• Treat symptoms with atropine I.V. • Temporary pacemaker or permanent pacemaker if considered for repeated episodes.
Wandering atrial pacemaker 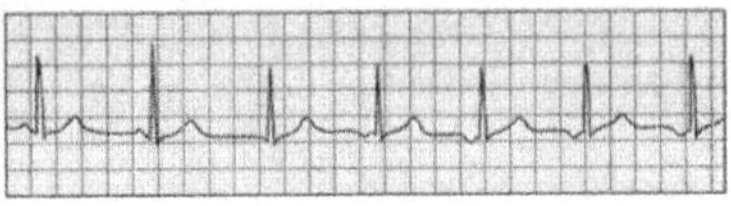	• Atrial and ventricular rhythms vary slightly. • Irregular PR interval. • P waves irregular with changing configurations indicating that they aren't all from SA node or single atrial focus; may appear after the QRS complex. • QRS complexes are uniform in shape but irregular in rhythm.	• Rheumatic carditis due to inflammation involving the SA node. • Digoxin toxicity • Sick sinus syndrome	• No treatment if patient is asymptomatic • Treatment of underlying cause if patient is symptomatic.
Premature atrial contraction (PAC) 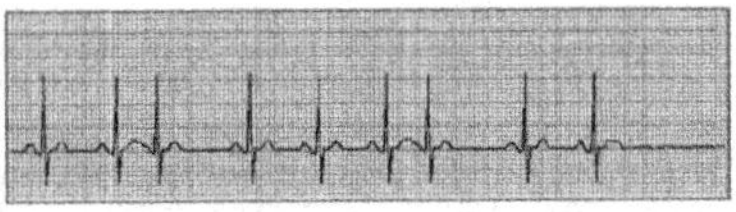	• Premature, abnormal-looking P waves that differ in configuration from normal P waves. • QRS complexes after P waves except in very early or blocked PACs. • P wave often buried in the preceding T wave or identified in the preceding T wave.	• May prelude supraventricular tachycardia. • Stimulants, hyperthyroidism, COPD, infection and other heart diseases.	• Usually no treatment is needed. • Treatment of underlying causes if the patient is symptomatic. • Carotid sinus massage. •

Cheat Sheet for ECG/EKG Interpretation

Arrhythmias	Description	Causes	Treatment
Paroxysmal Supraventricular Tachycardia 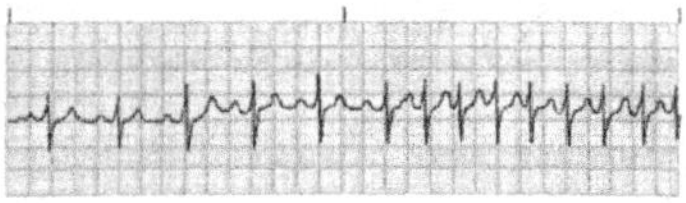	• Atrial and ventricular rhythms are regular. • Heart rate > 160 bpm; rarely exceeds 250 bpm. • P waves regular but aberrant; difficult to differentiate from preceding T waves. • P wave preceding each QRS complex. • Sudden onset and termination of arrhythmia • When a normal P wave is present, it's called paroxysmal atrial tachycardia; when a normal P wave isn't present, it's called paroxysmal junctional tachycardia.	• Physical exertion, emotion, stimulants, rheumatic heart diseases. • Intrinsic abnormality of AV conduction system. • Digoxin toxicity. • Use of caffeine, marijuana, or central nervous system stimulants.	• If the patient is unstable prepa for immediate cardioversion. • If the patient is stable, vagal stimulation, or Valsalva's maneuver, carotid sinus massa • Adenosine by rapid I.V. bolus injection to rapidly convert arrhythmia. • If a patient has normal ejection fraction, consider calcium chan blockers, beta-adrenergic block or amiodarone. • If a patient has an ejection fract less than 40%, consider amiodarone.
Atrial Flutter 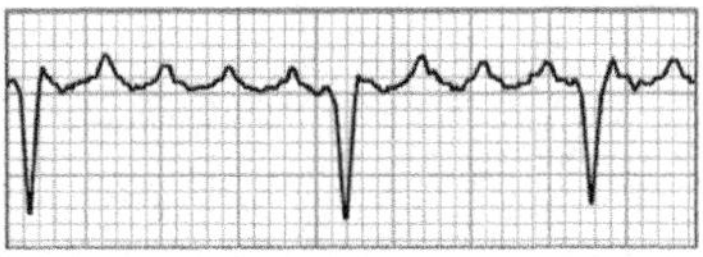	• Atrial rhythm regular, rate, 250 to 400 bpm • Ventricular rate variable, depending on degree of AV block • **Saw-tooth** shape P wave configuration. • QRS complexes are uniform in shape but often irregular in rate.	• Heart failure, tricuspid or mitral valve disease, pulmonary embolism, cor pulmonale, inferior wall MI, carditis. • Digoxin toxicity.	• If a patient is unstable with ventricular rate > 150bpm, prepare for immediate cardioversion. • If the patient is stable, drug therapy may include calcium channel blockers, beta-adrener blocks, or antiarrhythmics. • Anticoagulation therapy may be necessary.
Atrial Fibrillation 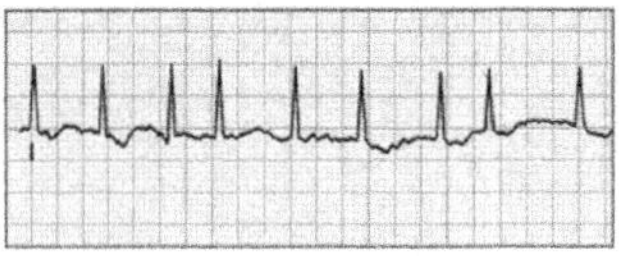	• Atrial rhythm grossly irregular rate > 300 to 600 bpm. • Ventricular rhythm grossly irregular, rate 160 to 180 bpm. • PR interval indiscernible. • No P waves, or P waves that appear as erratic, irregular base-line fibrillatory waves	• Heart failure, COPD, thyrotoxicosis, constrictive pericarditis, ischemic heart disease, sepsis, pulmonary embolus, rheumatic heart disease, hypertension, mitral stenosis, atrial irritation, complication of coronary bypass or valve replacement surgery	• If a patient is unstable with ventricu rate > 150bpm, prepare for immedi cardioversion. • If stable, drug therapy may include calcium channel blockers, beta-adrenergic blockers, digoxin, procainamide, quinidine, ibutilide, c amiodarone. • Anticoagulation therapy to prevent emboli. • Dual chamber atrial pacing, implantable atrial pacemaker, or surgical maze procedure may also b used.
Junctional Rhythm 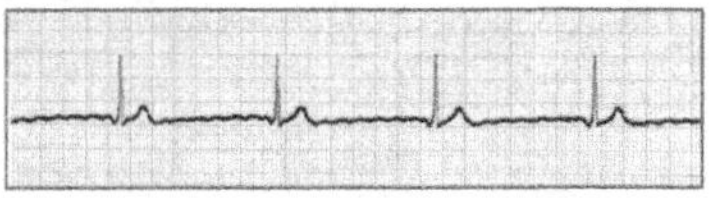	• Atrial and ventricular rhythms are regular. • Atrial rate 40 to 60 bpm. • Ventricular rate is usually 40 to 60 bpm. • P waves preceding, hidden within (absent), or after QRS complex; usually inverted if visible. • PR interval (when present) < 0.12 second • QRS complex configuration and duration normal, except in aberrant conduction.	• Inferior wall MI, or ischemia, hypoxia, vagal stimulation, sick sinus syndrome. • Acute rheumatic fever. • Valve surgery • Digoxin toxicity	• Correction of underlying cause. • Atropine for symptomatic slow rate • Pacemaker insertion if patient is refractory to drugs • Discontinuation of digoxin if appropriate.
Premature Junctional Conjunctions 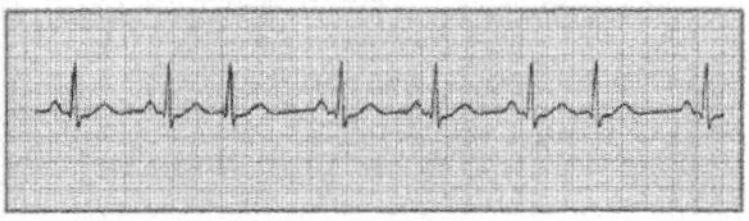	• Atrial and ventricular rhythms are irregular. • P waves inverted; may precede be hidden within, or follow QRS complex. • QRS complex configuration and duration normal.	• MI or ischemia • Digoxin toxicity and excessive caffeine or amphetamine use	• Correction of underlying cause. • Discontinuation of digoxin if appropriate.
First-degree AV block 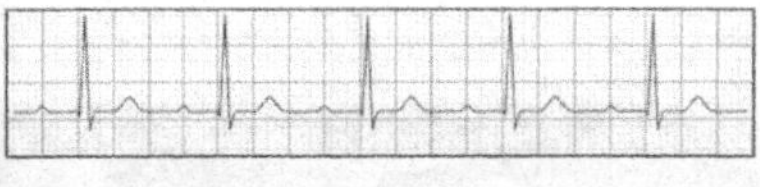	• Atrial and ventricular rhythms regular • PR interval > 0.20 second. • P wave preceding each QRS complex. • QRS complex normal.	• Inferior wall MI or ischemia or infarction, hypothyroidism, hypokalemia, hyperkalemia. • Digoxin toxicity. • Use of quinidine, procainamide, beta-adrenergic blocks, calcium	• Correction of the underlying cause. • Possibly atropine if PR interval exceeds 0.26 second or symptomatic bradycardia develops. • Cautious use of digoxin, calcium channel blockers, and zbeta-adrenergic blockers.

Cheat Sheet for ECG/EKG Interpretation

Arrhythmias	Description	Causes	Treatment
cond-degree AV block Mobitz I (Wenckebach) 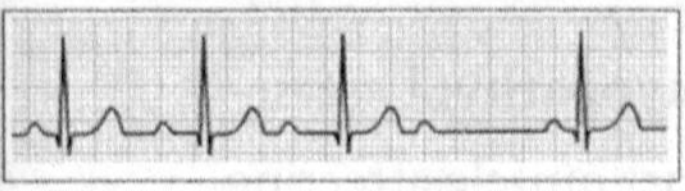	• Atrial rhythm regular. • Ventricular rhythm irregular. • Atrial rate exceeds ventricular rate. • PR interval progressively, but only slightly, longer with each cycle until QRS complex disappears. • PR interval shorter after dropped beat.	• Severe coronary artery disease, anterior wall MI, acute myocarditis. • Digoxin toxicity	• Atropine, epinephrine, and dopamine for symptomatic bradycardia. • Temporary or permanent pacemaker for symptomatic bradycardia. • Discontinuation of digoxin if appropriate.
hird-degree AV block (complete heart block) 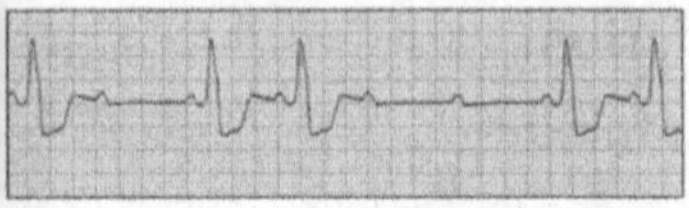	• Atrial rhythm regular. • Ventricular rhythm regular and rate slower than atrial rate. • No relation between P waves and QRS complexes. • No constant PR interval. • QRS interval normal (nodal pacemaker) or wide and bizarre (ventricular pacemaker).	• Inferior or anterior wall MI, congenital abnormality, rheumatic fever.	• Atropine, epinephrine, and dopamine for symptomatic bradycardia. • Temporary or permanent pacemaker for symptomatic bradycardia.
Premature ventricular contraction (PVC) 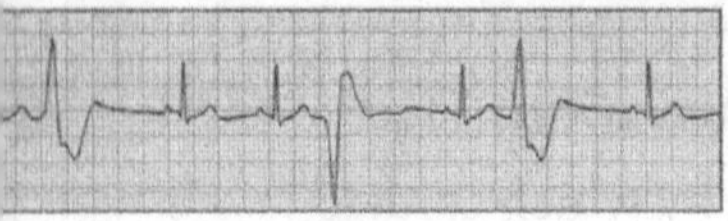	• Atrial rhythm regular • Ventricular rhythm irregular • QRS complex premature, usually followed by a complete compensatory pause • QRS complexes are wide and distorted, usually >0.14 second. • Premature QRS complexes occurring singly, in pairs, or in threes; alternating with normal beats; focus from one or more sites. • Ominous when clustered, multifocal, with R wave on T pattern.	• Heart failure; old or acute myocardial ischemia, infarction, or contusion. • Myocardial irritation by ventricular catheters such as a pacemaker. • Hypercapnia, hypokalemia, hypocalcemia. • Drug toxicity by cardiac glycosides, aminophylline, tricyclic antidepressants, beta-adrenergic. • Caffeine, tobacco, or alcohol use. • Psychological stress, anxiety, pain	• If warranted, procainamide, lidocaine, or amiodarone I.V. • Treatment of underlying cause. • Discontinuation of drug causing toxicity. • Potassium chloride IV if PVC induced by hypokalemia. • Magnesium sulfate IV if PVC induced by hypomagnesaemia.
Ventricular Tachycardia 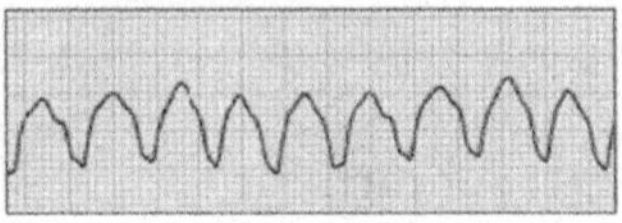	• Ventricular rate 140 to 220 bpm, regular or irregular. • QRS complexes wide, bizarre, and independent of P waves • P waves no discernible • May start and stop suddenly	• Myocardial ischemia, infarction, or aneurysm • Coronary artery disease • Rheumatic heart disease • Mitral valve prolapse, heart failure, cardiomyopathy • Ventricular catheters. • Hypokalemia, Hypercalcemia. • Pulmonary embolism. • Digoxin, procainamide, epinephrine, quinidine toxicity, anxiety.	• **If pulseless**: initiate CPR; follow ACLS protocol for defibrillation. • **If with pulse**: If hemodynamically stable, follow ACLS protocol for administration of amiodarone; if ineffective initiate synchronized cardioversion.
Ventricular Fibrillation 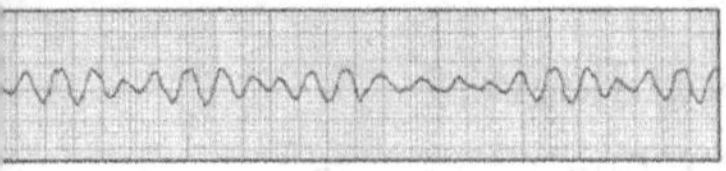	• Ventricular rhythm and rate are rapid and chaotic. • QRS complexes wide and irregular, no visible P waves	• Myocardial ischemia or infarction, R-on-T phenomenon, untreated ventricular tachycardia. • Hypokalemia, hyperkalemia, Hypercalcemia, alkalosis, electric shock, hypothermia. • Digoxin, epinephrine, or quinidine toxicity.	• **If pulseless**: start CPR, follow ACLS protocol for defibrillation, ET intubation, and administration of epinephrine or vasopressin, lidocaine, or amiodarone; ineffective consider magnesium sulfate.
Asystole 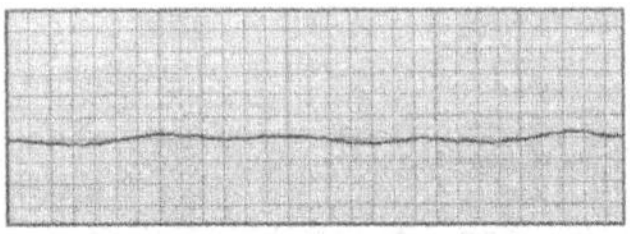	• No atrial or ventricular rate or rhythm. • No discernible P waves, QRS complexes, or T waves	• Myocardial ischemia or infarction, aortic valve disease, heart failure, hypoxemia, hypokalemia, severe acidosis, electric shock, ventricular arrhythmias, AV block, pulmonary embolism, heart rupture, cardiac tamponade, hyperkalemia, electromechanical dissociation. • Cocaine overdose.	• Start CPR.

GLOSSARY OF TERMS

Atrial Fibrillation (AFib): An irregular and often rapid heart rate originating in the atria.

Atrial Flutter: A rapid but regular rhythm originating from the atria.

Bradycardia: A slower than normal heart rate.

Bundle Branch Block: A blockage or delay in the pathway that electrical impulses travel to make the heart beat.

Cardiac Cycle: One complete heartbeat, including contraction and relaxation phases.

Cardiac Output: The volume of blood the heart pumps per minute.

Cardiomyopathy: Disease of the heart muscle affecting its size, shape, or structure.

Defibrillation: A treatment for life-threatening cardiac dysrhythmias using electrical shock.

Depolarization: The process by which cardiac muscle cells change their electrical charge, leading to contraction.

Ectopic Beat: A heartbeat originating outside the normal rhythm.

Electrocardiogram (ECG/EKG): A test that records the electrical activity of the heart.

Electrodes: Sensors placed on the skin to detect electrical activity.

Endocarditis: Inflammation of the inner lining of the heart chambers and valves.

Heart Block: A delay or complete block of electrical impulses from the atria to the ventricles.

Hyperkalemia: High levels of potassium in the blood, affecting heart rhythm.

Hypertension: High blood pressure.

Hypertrophic Cardiomyopathy: A condition where the heart muscle becomes abnormally thick.

Infarction: Tissue death due to inadequate blood supply, commonly referring to a heart attack.

Interval: The time between two specific points in the cardiac cycle on an ECG.

Ischemia: Reduced blood flow to tissues, leading to a lack of oxygen.

Lead: A specific view of the heart's electrical activity from the electrodes.

Left Axis Deviation (LAD): A deviation of the electrical axis of the heart to the left.

Myocardial Infarction (MI): Another term for a heart attack.

Myocardium: The muscular tissue of the heart.

Pacemaker: A device that regulates the heartbeat.

Palpitations: Sensations of a rapid or irregular heartbeat.

P Wave: Represents atrial depolarization on an ECG.

PR Interval: The time between the onset of atrial depolarization and the onset of ventricular depolarization.

PVC (Premature Ventricular Contraction): An early contraction of the ventricles.

QRS Complex: Represents ventricular depolarization on an ECG.

QT Interval: The time between the start of the Q wave and the end of the T wave.

Repolarization: The process by which cardiac muscle cells return to their resting electrical state.

Right Axis Deviation (RAD): A deviation of the electrical axis of the heart to the right.

SA Node (Sinoatrial Node): The natural pacemaker of the heart.

ST Segment: The flat, isoelectric section of the ECG between the end of the S wave and the start of the T wave.

Supraventricular Tachycardia (SVT): A rapid heart rate originating above the ventricles.

Syncope: Temporary loss of consciousness due to a drop in blood flow to the brain.

T Wave: Represents ventricular repolarization on an ECG.

Tachycardia: A faster than normal heart rate.

Torsades de Pointes: A specific type of abnormal heart rhythm that can lead to sudden cardiac death.

Tricuspid Valve: The heart valve between the right atrium and right ventricle.

U Wave: A small wave that follows the T wave on an ECG, sometimes seen in electrolyte imbalance.

Ventricular Fibrillation (V-Fib): A life-threatening heart rhythm that results in rapid, erratic electrical impulses.

Ventricular Tachycardia (V-Tach): A rapid heart rate originating from the ventricles.

Wenckebach Block: A type of second-degree heart block where the PR interval progressively lengthens until a beat is dropped.

Wolff-Parkinson-White Syndrome (WPW): A condition involving an extra electrical pathway in the heart.

Cardiomegaly: Enlargement of the heart.

Dysrhythmia: Another term for arrhythmia, an abnormal heart rhythm.

Electrophysiology: The study of the electrical properties of biological cells and tissues.

Holter Monitor: A portable device for continuously monitoring the electrical activity of the heart.

Heart Murmur: An unusual sound heard between heartbeats, often indicative of a valve problem.

Infarct: An area of dead tissue due to lack of blood supply.

Ischemic Heart Disease: A condition characterized by reduced blood supply to the heart muscle.

Lead I, II, III: Standard limb leads providing frontal plane views of the heart.

Left Bundle Branch Block (LBBB): A blockage in the left bundle branch of the heart's conduction system.

Multifocal Atrial Tachycardia (MAT): A rapid heart rate originating from multiple locations within the atria.

Paroxysmal: Sudden onset or sudden occurrence of symptoms.

Pericarditis: Inflammation of the pericardium, the fibrous sac surrounding the heart.

Prolonged QT Syndrome: A condition characterized by an extended QT interval on an ECG, predisposing to arrhythmias.

Pulmonary Embolism: A blockage in one of the pulmonary arteries in the lungs, often leading to heart strain.

Q Wave: The initial negative deflection in the QRS complex, sometimes indicative of myocardial infarction.

Sinus Arrhythmia: A normal variation in heart rate that occurs with breathing.

Sinus Bradycardia: A slow but regular heart rate originating from the sinoatrial node.

Sinus Rhythm: The normal regular rhythm of the heart set by the sinoatrial node.

Sinus Tachycardia: A fast but regular heart rate originating from the sinoatrial node.

ST Elevation: An upward deviation from the baseline in the ST segment, often indicative of myocardial infarction.

ST Depression: A downward deviation from the baseline in the ST segment, often indicative of ischemia.

Third-Degree Heart Block: A complete block of electrical impulses from the atria to the ventricles.

Trigeminy: A pattern of irregular heartbeats where every third beat is abnormal.

Vagal Maneuver: A technique used to slow the heart rate by stimulating the vagus nerve.

Vagal Tone: The level of activity of the vagus nerve, which can influence heart rate.

Vector: The directional flow of the electrical impulse through the heart.

Ventricular Bigeminy: A pattern of irregular heartbeats where every second beat is a PVC.

Ventricular Ectopy: Abnormal heartbeats originating from the ventricles.

Ventricular Septal Defect (VSD): A congenital hole in the heart's septum between the ventricles.

Waves: The graphical representation of the heart's electrical activity on an ECG.

Pacing: The use of a pacemaker to regulate heart rhythm.

Precordial Leads: Leads placed on the chest to record electrical activity from different angles.

Delta Wave: A slurred upstroke in the QRS complex, often associated with WPW syndrome.

Heart Rate Variability (HRV): The variation in time between each heartbeat.

Lown-Ganong-Levine Syndrome (LGL): A condition similar to WPW syndrome with an accessory pathway.

Ejection Fraction (EF): The percentage of blood pumped out of the ventricles with each heartbeat.

Fibrillation: Rapid and irregular contractions of the heart muscle fibers.

Intraventricular Conduction Delay (IVCD): A delay in the electrical conduction within the ventricles.

Non-ST Elevation Myocardial Infarction (NSTEMI): A type of heart attack that does not show ST elevation on an ECG.

Pulseless Electrical Activity (PEA): A condition where electrical activity is present on an ECG, but the heart is not pumping effectively.

Right Bundle Branch Block (RBBB): A blockage in the right bundle branch of the heart's conduction system.

Silent Myocardial Infarction: A heart attack that occurs without obvious symptoms.

Stress Test: A test to measure the heart's ability to respond to external stress in a controlled clinical environment.

Telemetry: Remote monitoring of a patient's heart rhythm.

Valsalva Maneuver: A breathing technique used to slow the heart rate.

Ventricular Hypertrophy: Thickening of the ventricular walls.

Biphasic P Wave: A P wave with both positive and negative components, indicating atrial enlargement.

Cardioversion: A medical procedure to restore a normal heart rhythm.

Electrocardiograph: The machine used to perform an ECG.

Hexaxial Reference System: A system used to determine the electrical axis of the heart.

Nodal Rhythm: A heart rhythm originating from the atrioventricular node.

Pre-excitation: Early activation of the ventricles due to an accessory pathway.

Sinus Arrest: A pause in the sinus rhythm due to the failure of the SA node to initiate an impulse.

Voltage Criteria: Measurements used to assess the amplitude of ECG waves for diagnosing conditions like hypertrophy.

FURTHER READING AND RESOURCES

Books

1. "The Only EKG Book You'll Ever Need" by Malcolm Thaler – A comprehensive guide suitable for both beginners and advanced learners.

2. "ECG Made Easy" by John Hampton – A simplified approach to understanding ECG interpretation.

3. "Rapid Interpretation of EKG's" by Dale Dubin – An easy-to-follow guide for quick learning of ECG basics.

4. "12-Lead ECG: The Art of Interpretation" by Tomas B. Garcia and Neil E. Holtz – A detailed book for mastering 12-lead ECG interpretation.

5. "Marriott's Practical Electrocardiography" by Galen S. Wagner and David G. Strauss – A thorough reference for advanced practitioners.

Online Courses

1. ECG Academy – Offers beginner to advanced courses on ECG interpretation.

2. Coursera: ECG Assessment: An Introduction for Healthcare Providers – A free course provided by Stanford University.

3. Udemy: Mastering ECG Interpretation – A course covering the essentials of ECG interpretation.

Websites

1. Life in the Fast Lane (LITFL) – A comprehensive online resource for ECG interpretation and emergency medicine.

2. ECG Library – A collection of ECG cases and tutorials.

3. American Heart Association (AHA) – Provides guidelines, articles, and resources on ECG and heart health.

Apps

1. ECG Guide by QxMD – A mobile app with a comprehensive ECG reference library.

2. Instant ECG – An app designed to teach and test your ECG interpretation skills.

Journals and Articles

1. Journal of Electrocardiology – Publishes research and reviews on electrocardiology.

2. Circulation: Arrhythmia and Electrophysiology – A journal from the American Heart Association focusing on arrhythmias and electrophysiology.

Practice Tools

1. SkillStat ECG Simulator – An online tool for practicing ECG interpretation.

2. ECG Quiz – Interactive quizzes to test your ECG knowledge and interpretation skills.

INDEX

A

B

F

G

H

I

J

L

M

N

P

Q

R

S

T

U

V

Made in the USA
Monee, IL
04 November 2026

67381190R00157